# MAN

# FELINE
# BEHAVIOUR

## Valerie O'Farrell
PhD

## Peter Neville
BSc (Hons)

Edited by
## Christopher St. C. Ross
BVM&S MRCVS

Published by the
British Small Animal
Veterinary Association,
Kingsley House, Church Lane,
Shurdington, Cheltenham,
Gloucestershire GL51 5TQ

Printed by J. Looker Printers,
Poole, Dorset.

The publishers and contributors cannot take any responsibility
for information provided on dosages and methods
of application of drugs mentioned in this publication.
Details of this kind must be verified by individual users
in the appropriate literature.

*First published 1994*

ISBN 0 905 214 24 2

# CONTENTS

636.8890

(2)

# CONTENTS

# AUTHORS

VALERIE O'FARRELL Ph.D.
**Department of Clinical Studies**
**Royal (Dick) School of Veterinary Studies**
**Edinburgh University**
**Summerhall Square**
**Edinburgh EH9 1QH**

Valerie O'Farrell graduated from Oxford University in 1963 in Psychology, Philosophy, and Physiology. She trained in Clinical Psychology at the Institute of Psychiatry, London and obtained a Ph.D. in Abnormal Psychology on the subject of ritualistic behaviour. She also trained in psychotherapy at the Tavistock Clinic, London. She held the posts of lecturer in the Department of Psychology, University College London and in the Department of Psychiatry, Edinburgh University. Since 1982 she has been attached to the Department of Veterinary Clinical Studies, Royal (Dick) School of Veterinary Studies, Edinburgh University as a Postdoctoral Research Fellow, where she provides a consultancy service for the owners of small animals with behavioural problems. Her research interests include the effect on dog behaviour of hormonal factors and of owner attitudes. Publications include the Manual of Canine Behaviour (1986, 1992), Problem Dog (1989) and Dog's Best Friend (1994).

PETER NEVILLE BSc. (Hons.)
**Bessant Neville Partnership**
**4 Quarry Cottages**
**Chicksgrove**
**Tisbury**
**Salisbury**
**Wiltshire SP3 6LZ**

Peter Neville graduated from the University of Lancaster in 1979 with a BSc. Honours degree in Biology. After spending three years with the Universities Federation for Animal Welfare working on the control and behaviour of feral cats, he joined an animal behavioural practice. In 1988 he set up a behavioural referral practice which still has clinics at Bristol Veterinary School. In 1992 he was awarded an honorary doctorate by the Etologisk Institute, Denmark, for studies of feline behaviour and the development of treatment for feline behavioural problems. He is currently Honorary Secretary of the Association of Pet Behaviour Counsellors and is the author of a number of books on pet behaviour problems including "Do Cats Need Shrinks?", "Claws and Purrs", and "Do Dogs Need Shrinks?".

# ACKNOWLEDGEMENTS

The task of editing this manual has been eased by the willing support and advice given by both Colin Price and Harvey Locke and by the fact that both authors worked to the suggested deadlines. In particular I would like to acknowledge the work Valerie O'Farrell has put into indexing and to Claire Bessant for her editorial expertise.

Thanks are also due to Claire Tickner for her secretarial and word processing skills, to Paul Worger of Foto Fantasia for his cover photograph, and to Russell Jones for his line drawings.

Finally I would like to thank the referring veterinary surgeons, their clients and patients who provided case material for this manual.

**Christopher St. C. Ross BVM&S MRCVS**

# FOREWORD

The companion volume to this new Manual, the Manual of Canine Behaviour, has proved to be very successful indicating the growing importance that behaviour problems have in veterinary practice. If one further considers the increase in the proportion of cats seen in the average small animal practice, the production of this new Manual is very timely.

Valerie O'Farrell and Peter Neville have ensured the information presented is in the same logical and easy to read format that has become the hallmark of the BSAVA Manual series. The success of treatment requires a good understanding of all the factors which influence behaviour in the domestic cat. Accordingly, the first section of the Manual has been devoted to an overview of these behavioural processes. The second half of the book deals with specific behaviour problems in more detail; using case histories where appropriate. Finally, consideration is given to the prevention of behaviour problems.

I am sure this format will make this new Manual as successful as its companion volume, and I would like to add my personal congratulations to the editor Chris Ross and authors for answering so many of the problems that are presented to the practitioner on a daily basis.

**Ray L Butcher MA VetMB MRCVS**
**President BSAVA 1993-94**

# INTRODUCTION

Chapter One

**The majority of veterinary surgeons are presented with many more behavioural problems in dogs than in cats**. There are various possible explanations for this. First, a cat's behaviour may be less likely to be problematic to its owner. It is, for example, much less likely to show dangerous aggression towards people. Second, owners usually expect dogs to conform to their wishes more than cats. For example, few cats are expected to obey commands or to go on walks or outings with their owners. Owners also tend to be more philosophical about behavioural lapses in their cats. When a dog steals food from the table, the owner is often enraged and filled with moral indignation; when a cat does the same, the owner is more likely to blame himself for having left it there.

Nonetheless, there is evidence that the issue is not so simple. A survey of the owners of 700 dogs and 800 cats (Voith, 1985) who had helped themselves to a questionnaire on display at a University Veterinary Hospital showed that 99% of both dog and cat owners regarded their pet as a family member. However, 47% of these cat owners considered that their cat engaged in some problem behaviour, as opposed to 42% of the dog owners. The situation probably also varies between cultures and countries and even regions.

**The difference in the frequencies of presentation to veterinary surgeons of behavioural problems in dogs and in cats may therefore be due not to a difference in their frequency of occurrence but rather to a greater willingness of dog owners to seek help**. This might be due to a more widespread expectation among dog owners that their pet's behaviour can and should be modified. Cat owners may be more tolerant of inconvenience caused by their pet's behaviour. In addition, they may simply be unaware that help is available. Veterinary surgeons might be well advised therefore to incorporate an enquiry about possible behavioural problems into routine health checks.

The commonest behavioural problem in cats is inappropriate urination or defecation. It accounted for 58% of 192 problems in a UK referral clinic (Neville, 1991) and for 24% of Voith's sample in the USA. In this latter study, destructive behaviour also accounted for 24% of the problems and ingestive behaviour problems for 20%. On the other hand, in the cases seen by Neville, aggression of various types was the next most common problem (16%). The increased frequency of presentation to a referral clinic of problems of inappropriate urination and defaecation and of aggression is presumably due to the greater disruption caused to a household by such problems.

**It seems likely that the number of behaviour problems in cats presenting to veterinary surgeons is going to increase in the future** given that cats are overtaking dogs in popularity (Messant & Horsefield, 1985). In particular the proportion of pedigree cats owned is increasing (Pet Food Manufacturers Association, 1992) and owners of these cats are more likely to seek help for problems. Neville (1991) found that although pedigree cats at the moment make up only 8% of the British pet cat population, they accounted for 44% of his referrals.

## THE STUDY OF CAT BEHAVIOUR

**Evidence from archaeology and alloenzyme studies (Randi & Ragli, 1991) point to the African wild cat (Felis sylvestris lybica) as the main ancestor of the domestic cat (Felis s. catus).** This conclusion is supported by behavioural evidence: the libyca sub-species is much easier to tame than the northern variety of the species, the Scottish wild cat (Felis s. sylvestris) (Serpell, 1988). Other more recent studies by Harley et al in South Africa (personal communication) using DNA mapping techniques have been unable to distinguish the domestic cat from the African wild cat while the European wild cat is clearly distinguishable from both. The implication is that the pet cat is genetically almost identical to the African wild cat. This is compatible with the fact that the earliest evidence of domestication is found in Egyptian paintings and effigies circa 2000 BC.

**Because the domestic cat has been subjected to less selective breeding than the domestic dog, its physical characteristics are more similar to its wild ancestor. The same is true of its behaviour.** For example, most cats are able to carry out a complete sequence of predatory behaviours: stalking, chasing, catching, killing and eating birds and small rodents. In most dogs, some parts of the hunting sequence are missing. Another consequence is that, although domestic cats do show individual and breed variation in temperament and behaviour (see Chapter 12), the variation in behaviour is much less pronounced than in dogs.

However, most serious study of this behaviour has been undertaken only comparatively recently. As a result of its convenience as an experimental animal, the cat has been extensively studied as a mammalian physiological system for over half a century, but much of the behavioural relevance of that physiology remains poorly understood. Detailed information is available about the cat's visual system and how information is processed in terms of movement, colour and binocular disparity, but the relevance of this system to, for example, a cat's predatory behaviour is still poorly understood.

In the same way, it is only in the past ten years that information about the cat's social organisation has become available. It used to be thought (Fox, 1974) that adult cats were by instinct asocial and that the attachment shown by a pet cat to its owner was a form of neotony i.e. juvenile behaviour persisting into adulthood. It is now known that adult cats do form cooperative social bonds with one another (see Chapter 3), although their communication system in terms of body, facial, scent and vocal language seems more subtle and less readily understood by owners than that of dogs.

The study of problem behaviour in cats also started later than in dogs. Again, this has happened despite the fact that when interest in experimental animal analogues of human neurosis was at its height in the 1940s and 1950s, some of the best known studies were carried out on cats (Masserman, 1943). However, in the past ten years, enough information has been gathered about cat behaviour and problem behaviour, its causes and treatment, to make systematic recommendations about the causes and effective treatment of problems.

## TREATMENT OF PROBLEM BEHAVIOUR

**It is a common misconception among veterinary surgeons, as well as pet owners, that**

**behaviour problems are more difficult to treat in the cat than in the dog**. However, follow-up studies indicate similar rates of response to treatment in both species. For example, in follow-up surveys carried out in the United States, 81% of cats with house soiling problems improved with treatment (Olm & Houpt, 1988), as compared with 82% of cats showing aggression redirected to people (Chapman & Voith, 1990). In a follow up survey of dogs treated for dominance aggression towards people, 88% were found to have improved (Line & Voith, 1986) and of dogs showing aggression towards other dogs outside the household, 75% had improved (O'Farrell, unpublished data). The reasons for this common misconception are instructive, however.

Dogs are by instinct pack animals, with most breeds and types expecting to live in a dominance hierarchy, and so it is relatively easy for an owner without special knowledge of dog behaviour to exert considerable control over their activities. The assumption that a dog is a furry human being will lead most owners to teach it desirable behaviour by means of praise and to dissuade it from undesirable behaviour by a dominant tone of voice and body language. These tactics are usually effective because most dogs are rewarded by social contact with pack members in the form of attention from the owner and because they expect to be controlled by dominant pack members. These anthropomorphic assumptions are, of course, inaccurate and problem solving tactics based on such premises sometimes fail. This has often happened in behavioural problems which come to the attention of veterinary surgeons or animal behaviourists. In these cases, such anthropomorphism, together with popular theories of "dog training", can be an impediment to successful treatment, as scientifically based recommendations may run directly counter to the owner's beliefs. When it comes to the treatment of cat behaviour problems, these impediments are usually not so great. Cat owners are, on the whole, less tempted to attribute human motives or human thought processes to their pets. They also tend to be less encumbered by false ideas about "cat training" and to have a lower expectation of being able to influence their pet's behaviour. Cat owners, therefore, tend to be more receptive to suggestions about possible treatment regimes and a behaviour consultant's job is thus made easier.

## ABOUT THIS BOOK

The aim of this book is to provide the veterinary surgeon with sufficient information to enable him or her to treat most cat behaviour problems. Some serious, complex or intractable cases, however, may still have to be referred to a specialist.

**The treatment of behaviour problems requires an understanding of all the factors which may influence an animal's behaviour. The first part of this book is therefore devoted to an overview of these behavioural processes. The second part deals with both common and unusual types of feline behaviour problem, their causes and treatment.**

# THE SENSES AND COGNITION

Chapter Two

Most owners are aware that their cats' senses are different from their own. One of their chief purposes is prey detection (see Chapter 3).

## VISION

Cats are naturally nocturnal or crepuscular hunters. However they will hunt during the day if the opportunity arises or if certain types of prey are more available (e.g. fledglings in spring). The eyes of the cat are well adapted for nocturnal vision: they are large with a pupil which can dilate widely, a reflective tapetum and a high proportion of cones to rods.

The cat, like other predators, has forward facing eyes to enable it to locate rodent prey. Each eye has a field of vision of 150-205 degrees, with 90-130 degrees overlap to produce binocular vision (Sherman, 1973). However, the cat cannot focus well on objects much closer than 75 centimetres, relying on its other senses when close to its prey. Its vision is optimum between two and six metres, when stalking small, fast-moving prey on the ground. Rodents may freeze if they suspect danger nearby; the cat may attempt to counter this by moving its head rapidly from side to side, which may improve its stereoscopic vision just before it pounces. Its eyes, which are best adapted to detecting movement, are thus enabled to pinpoint the prey and therefore gauge the final strike more accurately.

## HEARING

Cats can detect as great a range of sound frequencies (about 10.5 octaves) as any mammal (Fay, 1988) and they can detect high frequency sounds up to 85 kHz (Bradshaw, 1992) higher than either dogs or people. Cats are also better at locating the source of a sound because each pinna can be moved independently through more than 180 degrees. The abilities to detect high frequency sounds and to locate their sources are clearly useful when hunting rodent prey.

In the cat the semi-circular canals of the vestibular system are more nearly orthogonal than in other mammals (Wilson and Melville Jones, 1979). This endows it with a superior sense of balance and ability to right itself when falling.

## KINAESTHESIA

The whole body surface of the cat is sensitive to touch, but the long guard hairs, which stand slightly above the rest of the coat, are particularly sensitive. Movement of the hair gives the cat information about its immediate environment and also about wind direction; this is useful when the cat needs to approach prey from downwind. Kinaesthetic receptors are also concentrated in the pads of the paw.

On the other hand, cats are comparatively insensitive to heat, showing no reaction to a rise of body temperature to up to 52C caused, for example, by lying close to a fire (Kenshalo, 1964). They are, however, capable of detecting temperature differences of 0.5C via the skin of the nose. This is an adaptation which has become specialised and concentrated, like most other senses, in the face, with which the cat encounters most new environments first.

The carpal and cranial vibrissae help the cat to detect the proximity of objects close to the body. The carpal vibrissae are probably useful when catching prey (Nilsson and Skoglund, 1965). The position of the mystacial vibrissae (whiskers) varies with the cat's activity (Beadle, 1977): when it is walking, they project forward and laterally to scan a wide area. When the cat is sniffing or greeting, they are folded back close to the head.

## SMELL
The cat's olfactory bulb is relatively larger than ours: it contains about 67 million cells as compared with 52 million. Its sense of smell is therefore correspondingly keener, although inferior to that of the dog (Beadle, 1977). Cats almost certainly use airborne scent when detecting their prey. Rapid sniffing is used to investigate concentrations of smell or objects of particular interest via the Flehmen response (see page 14).

The newborn kitten has a well developed sense of smell which enables it to locate the mother's nipple (Rosenblatt, 1971).

Smell also plays an important role in communication. The adult cat uses its sense of smell to recognise other cats and probably other species as well. The development of a communal scent in a household must incorporate scent from the cat, its owners, other cats, other pets and from inanimate objects such as carpets and paint on doors. Many of these smells must contain the longer lasting fatty residues which the cat can discriminate so well. This is one of the reasons why it is important to incorporate the scent of any newcomers, especially babies or new cats, into the resident cat's scent environment as soon as possible.

Cats spend a great deal of time reinforcing the communal smell on their own bodies by rubbing members of the household and the furniture, to exchange scents. Owners usually sustain a successful scent relationship with their cats because they like to pet them and the cats enjoy it.

If a cat loses its sense of smell, for example because of a virus infection, it may become inappetent and its pattern of urinating behaviour may change. This is the basis for the suggestion that indoor spraying may be treated by olfactory tractotomy (see Chapter 10).

## TASTE
Tastebuds on the tongue are of little use in detection and capture of prey but they enable the cat to detect and recognise substances which dissolve in saliva once they have their teeth into their victims. Most cats show no response to sweetness, but they do respond to salt, bitter and acid tastes. They are very sensitive to the taste of water, which may account for bizarre individual preferences such as muddy puddles rather than clean but chlorinated water supplied by owners.

Like dogs and horses, cats possess an accessory olfactory organ: the vomeronasal or Jacobson's organ. They direct the scent laden air into it by means of a grimace referred to as the Flehmen response: the neck is stretched forward, the upper lip is raised and the mouth held open. Air is drawn in a series of short gasps and the tongue flicks back and forward over the two small openings behind the upper incisors. This dissolves the scent and directs it to the vomeronasal

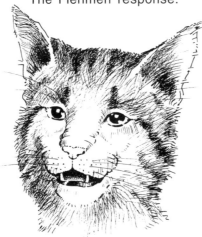

Figure 1
The Flehmen response.

organ. The Flehmen response seems to have a social function. It is typically seen in males during courtship and is also exhibited by both sexes while investigating urine marks.


## THINKING

Many canine behaviour problems are caused or compounded by the owner attributing human powers of thinking to the dog. On the whole, cat owners are less prone to this error. This is not necessarily because dogs are cleverer than cats. The measurement of animal intelligence and comparison between species is notoriously a problem, chiefly because it is difficult (and, many zoologists argue, inappropriate) to assess the contribution of the animal's innate biological capabilities to a particular piece of behaviour. For example, cats on the whole perform better than dogs at tasks which involve pulling strings and operating levers in a complicated sequence, because of their superior ability to perform fine manipulations with their paws. Dogs, on the other hand, tend to be better at tasks which involve obeying human commands, because of their innate ability to behave as subordinates in a dominance hierarchy.

In spite of such uncertainty, it is possible to be categorical about certain limitations to a cat's intelligence: these are not of merely theoretical interest. Although cat owners tend to be more realistic about their pets' mental powers than dog owners, they are still liable to over-estimate them, especially when upset by undesirable behaviour. An owner of a cat which sprays urine onto new curtains or defecates on the bed commonly interprets this as an act of spite by the cat or as revenge for some activity of the owner. **It is important for such owners to be clear about the limitation of their cats' thought processes, as such moral indignation is liable to interfere with the patient, methodical approach necessary for treating such problems.**

A cat cannot think abstractly or symbolically. It cannot ponder the past or make plans for the future. It is therefore useless for an owner to punish a cat for something it did even a few minutes previously, because the cat is incapable of making the connection between the action and the punishment. Conversely, its own actions can not be motivated by revenge for some past insult by the owner. By the same token, **a cat cannot understand the concept of a rule: it cannot follow rules or break rules**. House training, for example, is the result of a combination of classical conditioning (see below) and instinct (see Chapter 3) and not the result of conscientiousness or a sense of duty. Similarly, **a cat can have no notion of morality nor any idea of "right" or "wrong"**. Breakdowns in house training can be regarded neither as a dereliction of duty nor a deliberately spiteful response by the cat.

It is, however, also possible to underestimate a cat's cognitive abilities, a mistake made more often by scientists than by owners. In reaction against nineteenth century psychologists, who based their findings on introspection of their own thought processes, animal psychologists and ethologists during the first threequarters of this century insisted that only publicly observable events or actions were the proper objects of scientific study. An organism was regarded as a "black box": its input (stimuli) and output (responses) could be measured and relationships between the two worked out, but speculation about what went on inside the black box - i.e. thoughts - was fruitless. This mechanistic approach to animal behaviour (whose best known proponent was B. F. Skinner) led to useful generalisations about animal learning (see below). However, it also gave rise to the assumption that animals have no mental life: that they respond to their environment in an automatic, reflex way which is, in principle, entirely predictable. Evidence for the inappropriateness of this view will be discussed below, in the context of theories of learning.

Most owners have observed behaviour in their cats which is hard to explain purely on the basis of an association, learned or instinctive, between a stimulus and a response, but which is more easily explained in terms of mental process. For example, it is clear that many cats have a mental map of their home base and outdoor territory and that, when necessary, they can make their way from one point to another using a route they have never taken before.

Although it is clear that the generalisations of learning theory seriously underestimate the mental capabilities of mammals such as cats, they are nevertheless useful for explaining and attempting to alter learned behaviour patterns. There are two main types of learning: classical conditioning and instrumental learning.

## CLASSICAL CONDITIONING

This type of conditioning was first demonstrated by Pavlov in his famous investigations involving dogs. In the best known experiment, the dogs learned to salivate at the sound of a bell after being fed on several occasions when the bell was rung.

**Classical conditioning applies to involuntary or reflex responses (usually involving the autonomic nervous system). A reward for the behaviour is not necessary. A response becomes conditioned to a previously irrelevant stimulus, such as Pavlov's bell, if that stimulus is paired enough times with another stimulus which naturally or instinctively provokes the response.** Thus, in the case of Pavlov's dogs, the "unconditioned response" of salivation was naturally provoked by the "unconditioned stimulus" of the sight of food. The unconditioned stimulus was then paired with the "conditioned stimulus" of the bell and, eventually, that conditioned stimulus alone provoked the "conditioned response" of salivation.

For cat owners, the most relevant examples of responses which can be classically conditioned are concerned with elimination i.e. urination and defaecation. These responses are normally instinctively triggered by external stimuli such as the availability of a loose, easily raked substrate such as soil in a flower bed or litter in a tray (see Chapter 3). However, if for some reason the cat urinates or defaecates repeatedly on a different type of substrate, such as on a carpet or duvet, elimination may become conditioned to these less desirable substrates. Since classically conditioned responses are not maintained by a reward, a habit of inappropriate urination or defaecation once established, can continue indefinitely without any "motive", such as "revenge" or "attention-seeking". To treat such problems, it is necessary to re-condition the response of urination or defaecation to the appropriate stimuli (see Chapter 10).

Sexual responses, predatory behaviour and emotional responses such as fear or social aggression can also be classically conditioned (see Chapters 4, 8 and 9).

## INSTRUMENTAL LEARNING

In contrast to classical conditioning, **instrumental learning concerns voluntary actions and rewards**. If a stimulus prompts a response which is followed by a reward (technically known as reinforcement), when the animal encounters that stimulus again, the probability of it performing that response is increased . This general principle is constantly used in the training of dogs. For example, a dog may be taught to sit by giving the command "sit" (the stimulus) and, if this is followed by the dog sitting (the response), the owner rewards it with praise or a titbit (reinforcement). **Cats are as capable as dogs of instrumental learning, but few owners ever try to train them in the same way because it is not so immediately obvious what to offer a cat as a reward.** Most dogs find food or attention from their owners rewarding most of the time. Cats are less likely to be motivated by such prospects. However, with a little thought, appropriate rewards can be devised for cats; favourite food treats may be used, for example. As well as helping with problem behaviour, training by instrumental learning may make life easier and more interesting for both cat and owner. For example, cats can learn to retrieve objects; this can provide entertainment for the cat kept permanently indoors and helps to compensate for the lack of opportunity to stalk, chase and capture real prey. Outdoor cats can learn to mew or even to press a bell to be let in. All cats can relatively easily be taught to go to certain places and sit upright to "beg" for food at mealtimes.

On the other hand, **cats can also quickly learn less desirable behaviours**. They may learn to open a cupboard or container to help themselves to food, for instance. Sometimes the learned element has to be pointed out to the owner. A young cat which lies in wait to ambush people may initially be motivated by the need to play during the development of his predatory skills. However, the sudden movement, yells and flight of the victims may act as a reward and increase the intensity or frequency of the behaviour.

### Rewards
**Although food and social interaction are not as reliably rewarding for most cats as for dogs, they are rewarding some of the time for many cats. Other common rewards include: play, access to a favourite resting place and the opportunity to explore a new object.** Determining which experience might be rewarding for a particular cat at any particular moment usually requires sensitive observation on the part of the owner but many either observe their cats in this way already or are capable of doing so when they know what to look for. Behaviour problems in cats whose owners are unable or lack the motivation to observe them are always likely to be more difficult to treat.

For maximum impact, **a reward should be delivered at the same time as the response to be learned or immediately afterwards**. If the reward is delayed by even a second, the association with the response to be learned is weakened or other, undesired behaviour may be inadvertently rewarded. For example, in teaching a cat to sit up and beg, the food reward must be given as soon as the cat sits up. If the reward is delayed until the cat drops back down onto all fours, snatching the reward on the way, the snatch will be reinforced, not the begging position.

The frequency of reward is also important in determining the speed of learning. **A response is learned most quickly if it is rewarded every time it is performed correctly. But, once learned, a response is most resistant to unlearning (or extinction - see below) if it is then rewarded only intermittently and unpredictably.** When a new piece of behaviour is being taught, each correct response should be rewarded until the behaviour has been reliably learned. Only then can the proportion of correct responses which are rewarded be gradually reduced. By the same token, this may make some problem behaviour difficult to treat. Owners of vocal breeds such as Siamese may initially reward vocalisations with their attention. If the vocalisations become irritatingly frequent, owners may ignore them for as long as they can bear to, but occasionally they may feel forced to respond, thus maintaining the habit.

## Shaping

Owners sometimes need to teach their cats certain types of behaviour which they do not perform spontaneously, for example, learning to use a cat flap. Most owners soon abandon the method of physically forcing the cat into the required action when they discover that stuffing a cat through a cat flap is counter productive. **The best method of teaching a cat to use a flap is first to reward the cat for a response which it can be induced to perform spontaneously.** For example the flap may be wedged open and the cat called from the other side: when it joins the owner it is rewarded with a tit-bit and petting. The required response of pushing open a shut flap is gradually attained by repeating the process with the flap closed a little more each time the cat goes through it.

## Extinction

This term applies both to classical conditioning and instrumental learning. In classical conditioning, **extinction is the process by which a conditioned response becomes unlearned by repeatedly presenting the conditioned stimulus to the animal without the unconditioned stimulus.** Thus Pavlov's dogs eventually stopped salivating at the sound of the bell when they heard it on its own again and again without presentation of food. **Extinction also refers to the unlearning of an instrumentally learned response by ensuring that the learned behaviour is never subsequently rewarded.** Thus, if a behaviour is reinforced only by the reward of the owner's attention, it will eventually stop if the animal is consistently ignored when it performs that particular behaviour.

**When it is applicable and can be arranged satisfactorily, extinction is a reliable way of eliminating undesirable behaviour.** It is also safe, in that there is little risk of undesirable side effects unlike, for example, with the use of punishment (see below). Owners should be warned, however, that **once a response which has been reliably rewarded in the past is suddenly no longer rewarded, it may initially be performed with greater frequency than usual before its frequency gradually declines.** This is a phenomenon known as the "extinction burst" and owners who encounter this reaction unprepared may infer that the treatment plan is misguided and abandon the process of extinction before it has had a chance to take effect.

Extinction alone, however, is an inappropriate treatment for instrumentally learned behaviours where any repetitions of the behaviour are intolerable. Owners cannot wait for extinction to be effective when cats push ornaments off shelves to gain attention. In these cases, other techniques such as aversion must be used in addition to extinction programmes. Also, many classically conditioned responses, such as those involved in urination and defaecation problems or anxiety, are difficult to extinguish because other factors may cause the behaviour to become self perpetuating (see Chapters 3 and 4).

## Stimulus generalisation

Stimulus generalisation also applies to both classical conditioning and instrumental learning. It refers to a process whereby a response that has become conditioned to a certain stimulus will also be prompted by stimuli which are similar, but not identical, to the original stimulus. For example, a cat which has become conditioned to urinating on the sitting room carpet may, unless the problem is treated, gradually start urinating on other carpets in other areas of the house.

## PUNISHMENT

The first reaction of many cat owners to undesirable behaviour, such as inappropriate urination or stealing food from the kitchen table, is to punish their pet by smacking or shouting at it. Most cat owners, however, are more realistic than dog owners about the limitations of punishment. They soon discover, for example, that a cat smacked for jumping on a kitchen work surface may refrain from doing so in their presence but may continue to jump up when they are absent or out of range. Many owners still expect too much of punishment as a means of reforming undesirable behaviour. They often view it as the opposite of reward. The real opposite of reward is absence of reward i.e., extinction.

**Although punishment is sometimes successful in eliminating undesirable behaviour, it is less reliable and less safe than extinction** for various reasons. First, to be effective, **the intensity of the punishment must be exactly right**. If it is too strong, it may induce a state of fear in the cat which may last for some time. It may even provoke defensive aggression. If it is too weak, it will be ineffective at changing the undesirable behaviour. This difficulty cannot be circumvented by starting with a relatively weak punishing stimulus and gradually increasing the intensity, because repetition of any stimulus produces habituation: the recipient learns to tolerate the punishment. The cat which is continually shouted at ceases to be upset by it, even when the owner shouts ever more loudly. Also, it is not possible to make a standard recommendation about a suitable intensity of punishment. Different cats vary in their reactions to the same stimulus and even the same cat may vary in its reaction at different times. For example, a shout which is sufficiently alarming to deter it from sharpening its claws on the sofa may have no impact on its behaviour when it is crouched in the corner of the kitchen with a bird in its mouth.

Second, **it is clearly impossible to explain to a cat why it is being punished and so there is always a danger that it will associate the punishment with the wrong aspect of the situation.** Like rewards, punishments delivered even a second after the problem behaviour stand almost no chance of being effective. But even punishments delivered at exactly the right time may be misunderstood. An owner who smacks his cat when he catches it urinating indoors may teach it to urinate in another room away from him.

Third, **punishment tends to increase any animal's general level of anxiety**. If a problem is caused by anxiety in the first place (see Chapter 4), punishment is almost certain to compound the anxiety and make the problem worse. This often happens in cases of indoor urine spraying (see Chapter 10). In addition, other problems (such as certain cases of inappropriate urination) start for reasons other than stress (such as cystitis) and they may be aggravated by anxiety. In these cases, too, punishment is counter productive.

Occasionally punishment can be useful provided it is used carefully. **The risk of side effects is minimised if the punishing stimulus is mild**. It should simply startle or distract the cat from its actions. Examples of possible "punishing" distractions are a sudden, startling noise - a hiss is often particularly effective, presumably because it is similar to the noise that a cat makes when threatening a rival - or a surreptitious jet of water from a plant sprayer. Alternatively the punishment should be just sufficient to neutralise any rewarding effect of an undesireable behaviour. For example, the habit of chewing undesirable fabric or electric cables (as practised by some Siamese and Burmese cats in particular (see Chapter 11)) may sometimes be removed and the cat deterred by coating the items with an aromatic oil such as eucalyptus.

**An animal is more easily distracted from any behaviour when it is not highly motivated to perform it.** There is usually a point at the start of most activities when the motivation is comparatively low. For example, it is easier to distract a cat from sharpening its claws on a chair when it is walking towards the chair than when it has already started to scratch the material.

**Punishments or aversive events which seem to the cat to be "acts of God" are always preferable to those which are obviously carried out by the owner.** If the punishment is perceived by the cat to be caused directly by the undesirable behaviour it is more likely to refrain from the behaviour even in the owner's absence. There is also no risk of the punishment inducing a fear of the owner in the cat . Some apparent "act of God" punishments may be initiated by the owner at distance e.g. a water spray or an empty tin can thrown near the cat to make a startling clatter. An advantage of punishments initiated by the owner is that they can be delivered reliably and at exactly the right time. A disadvantage is that it is usually difficult for the owner to deceive the cat about the true origin of the punishment: it may soon learn the connection between the startling event and the owner. On the other hand, a booby trap (e.g. a pile of empty cans carefully balanced so that it collapses loudly when the cat jumps up on a kitchen work surface) may be less reliable in its operation but has the advantage of being truly unconnected with the owner.

**A punishment or distraction is always more effective if the animal is also provided with an alternative, rewarding action.** Thus, if a cat is distracted with a hiss from sharpening its claws on the sofa, it should be immediately be picked up, placed against a suitable scratching post and manually encouraged to make its scratching actions there.

## LIMITATIONS OF LEARNING THEORY

The foregoing generalisations about changing learned behaviour are based on learning theory. Since the 1970s, however, psychologists and ethologists have looked again at some of the assumptions on which the theory is based. For example, the validity of the distinction between instinctive and learned behaviour has been questioned. It has been pointed out, for instance, that **animals learn to perform new actions far more easily if they are similar to those already to be found in their instinctive behavioural repertoire:** a cat can easily learn to open a door with its paws because it uses a similar action when hooking a mouse out of the undergrowth. It is almost impossible, however, to teach a cat to open a door with its mouth.

Doubt has also been cast on the assumption that learning involves the animal making a connection between a stimulus and a response: that in order to learn a particular piece of behaviour, the animal must perform it. There are now various kinds of experimental evidence that this is not the case. The most relevant example for the pet owner is the observation that animals can learn to perform certain actions merely by watching their conspecifics (i.e. members of their own species). **Cats, for example, can learn to use a cat flap very quickly by watching others use it without having to employ their own "trial and error" approach or being taught by their owners.**

The most fundamental objection to learning theory, however, is that an animal cannot simply be viewed as a machine (such as a hot drinks dispenser) which passively receives a stimulus (e.g. the push of a button) that automatically triggers a response (e.g. a cup of coffee). Experiments have only recently started to demonstrate what every pet owner knows - that every cat or dog chooses which are the important stimuli to be attended and responded to and which are irrelevant and to be ignored. Anyone who has tried to train a dog knows that there is no point in giving a command unless he first has the dog's attention. Most recent models of animal behaviour and learning incorporate the assumption that **an animal is actively engaged in gathering information about his environment and trying to predict what will happen in it**. Such models, however, have yet to generate either such simple or such useful laws about how animals learn as the older models of animal behaviour and learning do.

## FURTHER READING

BEAVER B. V. (1992). *Feline Behaviour: a Guide for Veterinarians*. W. B. Saunders, Philadelphia

BRADSHAW J. W. S. (1992). *Behaviour of the Domestic Cat*. Wallingford. CAB International. Chapters 2 and 3

BORCHELT P. L. and Voith V. L. (1985). Punishment. *The Compendium on Continuing Education for the Practicing Veterinarian*. **7**: 780-788.

NEVILLE P. (1992). *Claws and Purrs*. Sidgewick and Jackson, London.

# INSTINCTIVE BEHAVIOUR

## Chapter Three

Although the instinctive behaviour patterns of the domestic cat have survived in a more complete form than those of the dog, they are less well understood. This is partly due to the fact that less attention has been paid to cats but work in recent years has started to rectify the balance.

## SOCIAL BEHAVIOUR

**It used to be thought that cats were solitary creatures which, once adult, sought the company of their own species only for the purposes of mating and breeding. However, it is now recognised that some feral cats voluntarily form colonies with high levels of social interaction.** Similarly, a questionnaire survey of the owners of 500 pet cats in the USA (Voith and Borchelt, 1986) found that 71% of cats in multi-cat households frequently played with each other, 66% slept together and 58% groomed each other. Factors which influenced the tendency towards sociability seem to be:

1.  Availability and dispersion of food: feral cats which support themselves by hunting prey dispersed over a wide area tend to lead solitary lives. When there is an abundant food source concentrated at one point (e.g. when a cat lover regularly puts out food) a relatively stable group of cats tends to form around it (Kerby and Macdonald, 1988). The same applies to pet cats attached to one household.

2.  Shelter: feral cat colony size is sometimes governed by the availability of suitable shelter positions rather than by the availability of food (Bradshaw, 1992). Except, perhaps, for households keeping large numbers of cats, pet cats normally find shelter easily.

3.  Gender: most feral cat colonies consist of related females and their offspring. New members are recruited to the group by birth – strange females usually being excluded. Mature males are usually more loosely attached to several groups and often move between different groups of fertile females. Neutering mature male feral cats seems to result in little change in their social behaviour, but there is some evidence (Bradshaw, 1992) that neutering immature males before they leave the group may freeze their behaviour at that more sociable stage, maintaining their bonds with their mother and other females in her group.

4.  Personality: some cats seem to be more tolerant of the presence of conspecifics than others. The origins of this type of personality difference are not yet fully understood, but both genetic

and early environmental influences are probably important. Owners who want to keep two or more cats in their household cannot be certain that all of their cats will co-exist amicably. However, they can maximise the chances of this by acquiring female litter mates as kittens or males which are castrated before puberty. If possible, the kittens should be of a mother which is on friendly terms with the other cats in her own household. The problem of introducing a new cat into a household where a cat is already established is dealt with on page 72.

Cats which have had sufficient contact as kittens with human beings behave similarly towards them as they would towards conspecifics (see Chapter 5). However, sociability with people is a separate personality trait not correlated with sociability with other cats. Owners who want to maximise their chances of obtaining a sociable cat should look for a kitten with the appropriate early experience (Chapter 5) and whose mother is sociable with people. Hence most kittens born to a 'pet cat' mother and raised in a normal domestic household usually make sociable friendly pets.

The social structure of cat groups is not yet fully understood. There seems to be some group cooperation, particularly among females who may share the rearing of each others' kittens ( Macdonald *et al* 1987). A cat may also have a preferred partner within the group, although this preference is apparently not always mutual (Bradshaw, 1992). **Cat groups do not seem to establish a clear dominance hierarchy in the same way as wolves or most dogs.** Although an individual cat in a group may have precedence in access to resources such as food, such precedence does not seem to be claimed by displays of dominance nor acknowledged by displays of submission by other cats as in dog or wolf packs. Instead, when provoked, the 'superior' cat may show actual aggression or pronounced threat behaviour towards the others to which they respond with defensive or fearful, rather than appeasing, behaviour (Voith and Borchelt, 1986).

A cat signals a friendly approach to another with a body posture which is characterised by a slightly raised tail (see figure 2). Friendly pairs of cats will then groom each other. They will also rub their heads and flanks together both to achieve familiarity through touch and to exchange scent from glands on the face and from the fur. Rubbing seems to be more frequent in one sided relationships with the cat seeking the interaction being the one which initiates the rubbing.

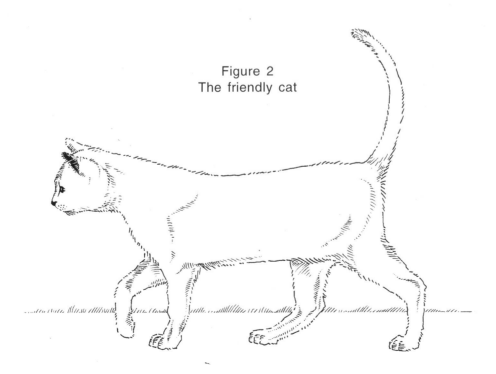

Figure 2
The friendly cat

Figure 3
The confident cat

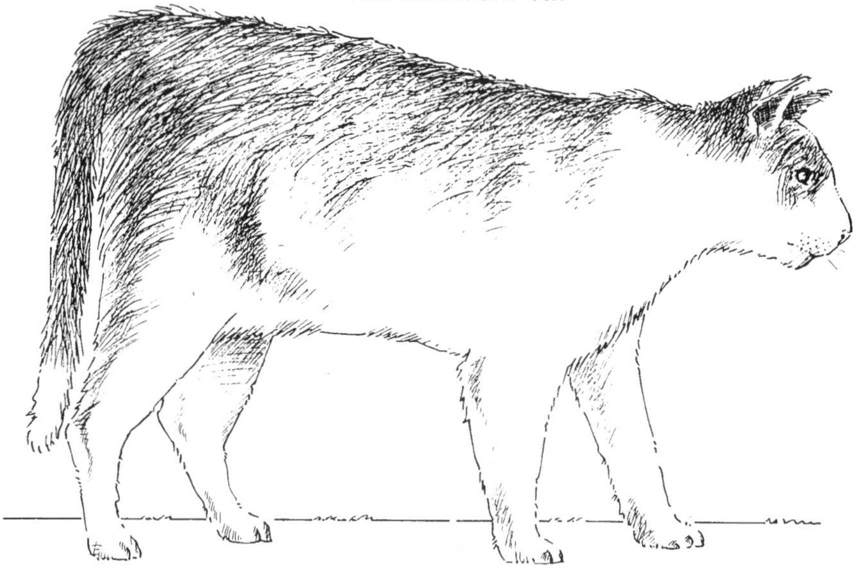

A cat which is confident approaches its opponent head-on; its fur may be erect and it draws itself up to its full height, with the hind quarters raised. The ears are pricked and turned forwards (see figure 3). A cat which is fearful or defensive may try to reduce its size by crouching on the ground with its coat and ears flattened (see figure 4a). Alternatively, it may adopt the more dramatic posture shown in figure 4b. The cat stands sideways on to its opponent, with ears flattened but fur standing on end, back arched and tail erect.

Most owners understand their cat's body language well, at least with regard to friendly behaviour. They recognise that when their cat rubs against them or licks their hand it is being affectionate. However, **cat owners may suffer from the fact that the special preferences that cats may adopt in social group are not always mutual and, as a result, they may not enjoy as close a relationship as they had hoped for.** A cat's choice of favourite person in a household may seem perverse when a cat chooses a family member who has little affection for it. A study by Turner (1991) sheds some light on this phenomenon. Analysis of the interaction between 158 cat owner pairs showed that the more interactions which were initiated by the owner, the less the total interaction time they enjoyed together. In other words, **a cat spends more time with its owner if it, rather than the owner, takes the initiative in these interactions.** Thus, the cat-loving member of a household may spoil his or her relationship with the cat by approaching it too frequently prompting it to prefer another member of the family who ignores it and with whom it can control the relationship more effectively. These findings would come as no surprise to most experienced cat owners, who know that the way to build a good relationship with a cat is not to force your attentions upon it but to respond to its social initiatives. Further findings from the study by Turner confirm this: owners who were more responsive to their cats' overtures were more likely to have cats which responded to them in return.

## TERRITORIAL BEHAVIOUR

**Cats are territorial animals. The territory of indoor cats consists of the house; for outdoor cats, it extends to the surrounding gardens and streets and maybe beyond.** Outdoor territories usually overlap the territories of other cats. The cats may compete and fight over access to resources in the area or reach a sort of time-sharing agreement (Leyhausen, 1965). More assertive cats can move unopposed at any time. They enforce their right to do so by attacking other cats at important times of day such as the evening when rodents become active. Meeker individuals may only be allowed to use the territory at less desirable times of day, such as midday, when prey

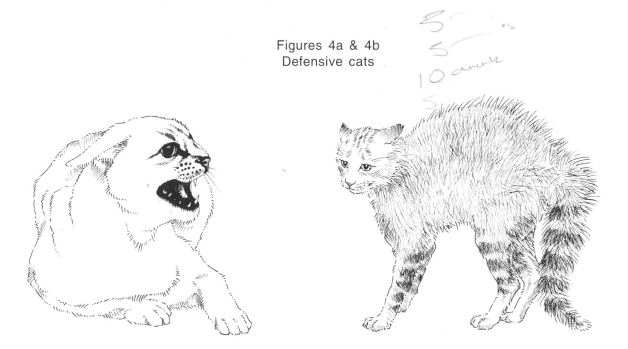
Figures 4a & 4b
Defensive cats

is scarcer. Males, especially entire toms, tend to have larger territories than females.

**Cats scent mark their territories in various ways. The most easily recognised is urine spraying**. Sprayed urine usually contains glandular secretions as well as urine: it probably conveys information to other cats about the sprayer's gender, age, hormonal state and general health (Bradshaw, 1992). Cats can also judge how recently a spray mark was made. **Faeces is also sometimes used for marking, a behaviour known as middening.** Cats normally bury their faeces but, when middening, they leave it deliberately exposed. They do this mostly in areas of their territory under challenge, especially by other cats or other species which mark similarly, such as foxes. Middening occasionally occurs indoors as well (see page 63).

**Claw sharpening on vertical surfaces such as trees or furniture is often also a territory marking behaviour:** it provides both a visual signal and an olfactory one, with scent deposited by pedal glands during the action of clawing. In addition, the secretions of the submandibular cheek and perioral glands are deposited on projections such as twigs in anointing behaviour known as bunting.

The function of these various forms of territorial marking is as yet imperfectly understood. It must be at least partly to deter neighbouring cats or at least keep them at a comfortable distance. For entire males and breeding females, urine spraying must also provide important information about potential mates and rivals. Claw sharpening frequently occurs in the presence of conspecifics and may constitute some form of threat or display of confidence. As well as being deposited on twigs, head gland secretions are exchanged with that of conspecifics during affectionate rubbing: they probably help to develop a communal or shared scent for each cat and so generate a feeling of group solidarity. Most forms of marking may provide a feeling of comfort and security for the perpetrator, rather like spreading one's possessions around a strange hotel bedroom. Feral cats may spray urine throughout their hunting range and even at the core of their territory, which is not always under threat by other cats. Similarly, a new cat trying to join a feral colony may enter the feeding area at quiet. non-feeding times and spray, bunt and midden to announce his intention to join the group (Tabor, 1983). When he does finally introduce himself to the other cats, their hostility will be reduced by their familiarity with his smell. **Indoor spraying in pet cats may be triggered by the arrival of a new cat, dog or person in the family or even by the appearance of new objects.**

## HUNTING

Unlike the domestic dog, the domestic cat is usually a competent predator, foraging from home despite being fed prepared food there. It hunts and kills small prey, chiefly rodents and garden birds. Some learning is necessary for the development of hunting skills and, for most cats, this takes place when they are kittens (see chapter 5). However, cats which miss out on the appropriate learning at this stage, perhaps through lack of opportunity, usually manage to catch up later by practicing on their own.

Providing a cat with adequate food does not abolish predatory behaviour, as most owners of outdoor cats discover. There is no conclusive evidence that feeding even reduces hunting, although feral cats spend a greater proportion of the day hunting than their pet counterparts. Cats have two main hunting strategies, patrolling and ambushing. They either walk through their hunting range listening and looking for promising sights and sounds or they sit and wait quietly at an area where they have enjoyed success before, usually by a rodent burrow, and wait for the opportunity to strike. Their attention is particularly attracted by movement and high-pitched sounds (such as a rodent's squeak) which the cat's hearing has evolved to detect. Most experienced cat owners understand these aspects of cat behaviour intuitively and use them in play with their cats. For example, after exciting the cat to a state of anticipation by making rustling, squeaking or scratching sounds, they may dangle a toy mouse from behind an object; or they may make it shoot suddenly across the floor in a way which mimics the jerky actions and fast movements of a small live rodent. Owners usually enjoy playing with their cats in this way, although they may not realise that they are helping it to practice and improve its hunting skills.

While most owners of outdoor cats accept that their cat cannot be dissuaded from hunting and killing their natural prey, many are upset when their cat does not kill its prey immediately, but repeatedly releases and recaptures it. It is possible that this behaviour, which owners often interpret as sadistic teasing, arises from a failure to learn how to kill the prey with the characteristic nape bite of cats. Hence, as long as the animal can escape and continue to move, it will excite the cat's stalk and chase behaviour. If, in the process of exercising its capture techniques, the cat frightens or batters the victim to death, it finally loses interest in the body or is distracted by the next moving target. There is also evidence (Biben, 1979) that playing with prey rather than killing and eating it may be a form of displacement activity (see Chapter 4). This might result from a conflict between a desire to kill the prey and fear of the injury which it might inflict on an inexperienced hunter.

Figure 5
The hunting cat

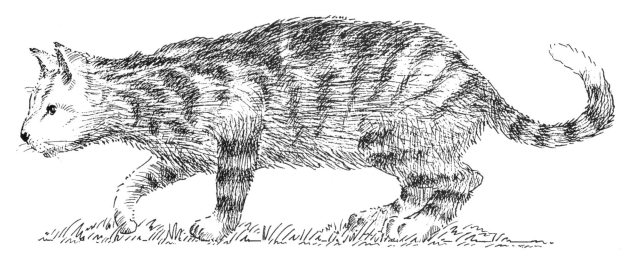

# CATS AND THE VETERINARY CONSULTATION

In approaching an unfamiliar cat, veterinary surgeons should try to mimic the greeting behaviour of a friendly cat to an unfamiliar cat. As cats in this situation greet each other by extending their necks to sniff, the veterinary surgeon should get down to the cat's level and approach it slowly face to face. He can do this most easily by placing the cat, probably still in its carrying basket, on a raised examination table. He should half close his eyes and blink, rather than staring which is often interpreted by cats as a threatening expression. Sudden arm movements, particularly from above, should not be used, as the cat may perceive these as threatening. When the cat stretches its neck and head forward to sniff, he may slowly extend his hand towards it. The hand should then be slowly put into the basket and used to rub the cat's head and chin prior to more invasive handling or gentle removal from the basket.

Veterinary surgeons who feel they are at risk of being bitten by a dog during a consultation may adopt the tactic of speaking to it fiercely or even hitting it in an attempt to force it into a subordinate role. This is a risky enough tactic to employ with dogs, but with cats it is certain to be counter-productive. A cat showing the body posture of figure 4a (page 23) is not indicating submission, but is on the defensive, and will become aggressive if further threatened.

## FURTHER READING

BRADSHAW J. W. S. (1992). *Behaviour of the Domestic Cat.* CAB International. Wallingford. Chapters 5,7 and 8.

TURNER D. C. and Bateson P. (Eds) (1988) *The Domestic Cat: The Biology of Its Behaviour.* Cambridge University Press. Section 3.

VOITH V. L. and Borchelt P. L. (1986). Social Behaviour of Domestic Cats. *The Compendium on Continuing Education for the Practicing Veterinarian.* **8**, 637-644.

# ANXIETY AND STRESS

Chapter Four

In order to survive, any animal must be able to respond to his environment with an appropriate level of arousal. It must be able to rest calmly when nothing in particular is going on, but respond with a high level of arousal if something occurs which calls for action. In man, such high levels of arousal, extended over a long period, can lead to problems, both psychological and physical. The same is true of other animals, including cats.

## FEARS AND PHOBIAS

When threatened, cats, like most mammals, have four major defence strategies:- withdrawal (flight from the threat), immobility (crouching and lying still to avoid attracting attention), deflection/ appeasement (actively submitting to the attacker) and defensive aggression.

When a cat crouches down with ears flattened back, or runs away or hides, it is obvious to most owners that it is afraid and adopting the first or second of these strategies. In contrast to dogs, fearful cats rarely attempt to appease threatening challenges. Occasionally, however, female cats in particular may roll over to expose the abdomen engaging in mock forms of mate solicitation in an effort to deflect a threat from another cat.

Owners sometimes make mistakes in the interpretation of the their cat's body language when it is fearful. For example, a defensive posture of crouching immobility may be mistaken for an impending aggressive attack because it looks similar to the stalking crouch used by the cat when hunting (see page 24). In reality, the fearful cat is most unlikely to attack from the immobile position unless it is further threatened, although the nature of the threat may not be obvious to the owner. For example, a fearful cat may attack an innocent bystander as a form of redirected aggression (see page 49).

Some fears, such as fear of a moving car, are essential for a modern pet cat's survival in the town. Others, for instance, fear of a particular person in the household, may be maladaptive and, when extreme, such fears are termed phobias. **Some phobias seem to be partly caused by an innate sensitivity.** For example, cats often react with fear to their first contact with a snake. This behaviour has presumably evolved because of its survival value. Most mammals, including cats, also fear new and strange sights or sounds. Sensitivity to novelty varies throughout life: it is at its lowest during the later stages of weaning when necessary exploratory behaviour can be supervised by the parents.

**Many phobias contain a learned component.** This may arise from a single unpleasant experience. For example, Kertsin (1968) presented a hungry cat with an electrified mouse, which delivered a 4V shock when the cat pounced on it. The result was that for weeks afterwards the cat was afraid of mice. The painful or unpleasant stimulus (such as the shock) evokes unconditioned responses of the autonomic nervous system. These responses then become conditioned to the sight of the mouse. For the pet cat, a similar process can occur when it is restrained and pills are forced down its throat. The result may be that it subsequently runs into the garden whenever the bottle of pills is produced.

The conditioned fearful response may then also generalise onto similar stimuli such as the sight or sound of other small plastic containers. This process was experimentally demonstrated by Wolpe (1952) who induced a phobic reaction in cats by putting them in experimental cages and administering electric shocks. Subsequently, the closer the resemblance of the cage that the cats were housed in to the experimental cage, the greater was the intensity of their fearful reaction.

Classically conditioned responses tend to extinguish when the conditioned stimulus appears repeatedly without the unconditioned stimulus. Thus most baseless fears tend to become unlearned in the normal course of events. Why a few such fears do not extinguish and go on to become established as phobias is not entirely clear. If the unconditioned stimulus is highly traumatic, then the associated conditioned stimuli may, on their own, continue indefinitely to provoke a fear response. For example, Solomon and Wynne (1963) carried out an experiment in which dogs first heard a buzzer and then received a near-fatal electric shock, which they could only escape by jumping over a barrier. After this experience, the dogs always jumped the barrier whenever they heard the buzzer, even though it was never again paired with a shock of any kind over hundreds of trials.

It seems likely that cats sometimes acquire phobias in this way, for example when injured by a car. Most phobias, however, start with a much less traumatic experience and cannot be explained in this way. In these instances, it seems likely that the experience of the fear reaction itself is so unpleasant that it operates thereafter as an unconditioned stimulus. For example, people who suffer from a phobia of lifts usually do not need an unpleasant external event, such as the lift getting stuck, to maintain their fear. The internal events of pounding heart, cold sweat, breathlessness etc, that occur every time they take a trip in a lift are enough to perpetuate the phobic reaction.

**A phobia, therefore, cannot be cured by the "commonsense" method of exposing the sufferer repeatedly to the feared situation** in the hope that it will realise that its fears are groundless. If a cat which is phobic of visitors is introduced to everyone who calls, it will probably continue to run away and hide every time. **A phobia can, however, be unlearned if the behavioural method known as systematic desensitization is employed.** This involves exposing the animal only to versions of the feared stimulus which are so mild that little or no anxiety is provoked. The intensity of the stimulus is then increased in gradual stages until, finally, the level of the stimulus which originally provoked the phobic reaction can be presented without inducing massive anxiety. This process of desensitization is helped if the cat's background anxiety level is as low as possible when the anxiety provoking stimulus is presented. This is best achieved by first relaxing and distracting the cat through feeding or petting or, if other methods fail, by means of anxiety-reducing drugs (see pages 42-43). This method can also be used in the treatment of problems which involve other kinds of learned emotion, such as certain forms of aggression.

## STRESS REACTIONS

Stress reactions are commonly provoked by a threatening situation which cannot be dealt with by flight, immobility, appeasement or aggression. Situations which cause stress in cats are:

1.  **Territorial invasion**
    **A cat's security may be threatened if its house or home range of garden or street is**

**invaded** by new cats, people or other animals. Some may show symptoms of stress. **It may also be stressed if moved to new surroundings.** For example, many cats are less upset if they are left alone at home when their owners go on holiday, with a neighbour calling in to feed them, than if they are boarded in a cattery.

2. **Punishment**

As discussed on page 18 punishment can produce a learned fear reaction to stimuli associated with it. Although this kind of specific effect on a cat's behaviour is often the aim of owners who use punishment, it may also give rise to more general and undesirable stress reactions. For example, Masserman (1943) taught cats to operate a switch to obtain a pellet of salmon. He then gave them an electric shock or a blast of air in the face as they took the pellet. In addition to developing a fear of the apparatus, some of the cats also began to show signs of stress outside the experimental situation. Although the presence of additional features, such as confinement, uncertainty or conflict (see below) makes the development of generalised stress reactions more likely, their appearance or intensity cannot be predicted with certainty in any one individual. As explained on page 18, this is one of the reasons why punishment is best avoided in trying to treat behaviour problems.

3. **Confinement**

Confinement or restraint is stressful for most animals and this is certainly true for cats: a fact which is brought home to many owners when they transport their cats in a basket or cage. Therefore, when recommending caging as part of a treatment regime (for example, of intolerance of another cat in the household, see page 47), it is important to check that this measure is not itself producing additional stress.

4. **Conflict and uncertainty**

Many animal experiments have demonstrated that conflict produces anxiety, especially if the animal is at once attracted to, yet frightened by, the same thing. This leads to an approach/avoidance conflict. When Masserman punished his feeding cats, he must have produced this kind of conflict. **In pet cats as well as dogs, one of the commonest kinds of approach/avoidance conflict is attachment to the owner accompanied by fear.** This fear may be the result of the owner shouting at or punishing the animal unpredictably or repeatedly.

Making a difficult decision or discrimination is another kind of conflict which may produce anxiety. This was demonstrated in an experiment by Thomas and DeWald (1977) in which cats were presented with a light and a dark coloured lever. Pressing the light coloured lever was rewarded with food but pressing the dark one was not. When the cats had learned this reliably, the dark lever was progressively lightened until it was the same shade as the light lever. At this point, the cats became agitated and aggressive; they eventually stopped pressing any levers and sat or lay immobile, in fixed postures which are often characteristic of stress (see below). For some pet cats, a common source of this type of uncertainty is disruption of the general domestic routine, for example during school holidays. Also, **if the cat is particularly attached to a family member, it may be stressed if that person starts to behave inconsistently towards it**, during a period of their own emotional instability.

5. **Personality**

Experienced cat owners know that cats show individual variation in their general behaviour, sensitivity and reactions to stress. Several investigations (Feaver et al, 1986; Karsh & Turner, 1988; Mendl, 1990) have demonstrated two relevant dimensions of personality which can be reliably assessed by observer ratings or measured by performance in behavioural tests. **A cat may be either equable and easy going or reactive and nervous. It may also be either outgoing and sociable or aloof and reserved.** These dimensions seem similar to those first described by Pavlov (1927) in the dog and to those later described in people by Eysenck (1960). He described human personality using the dimensions of "neuroticism" and "introversion/

extraversion". He also suggested that the position of neurotic individuals on the introversion/ extraversion dimension determined the type of the neurotic symptoms from which they suffered. Introverts tend to suffer from phobias or obsessional symptoms while extraverts are more likely to engage in hysterical, antisocial or self-destructive behaviour. The same may apply to cats (see below).

**There is evidence that early environment can have an effect on both a cat's sociability and its nervousness** (see Chapter 5). There is also evidence for a genetic influence on these parameters in both dogs and man. Similarly Turner (1986) found that the friendliness of kittens was significantly affected by the friendliness of their fathers, with whom they had never come into contact. The generally accepted personality differences between cat breeds are additional evidence for a genetic influence: Siamese and Burmese are often extraverts, Rex cats tend to be more neurotic and Persians are more likely to be placid introverts. (For further discussion of breed differences, see page 71).

## MANIFESTATIONS OF STRESS

**Some manifestations of stress are more cryptic than others.** It is usually obvious to owners when an extraverted cat is generally nervous or reactive but an introverted cat may be withdrawn and immobile, sitting in a fixed posture which goes un-noticed. A common reaction to stress in cats is an increase in territorial marking outdoors, perhaps prompted by the challenge of a new cat in the locality, or indoors due to the acquisition of a dog by the family.

**Displacement activity is also a common response to emotional conflict.** This may consist of entire instinctive behavioural sequences (such as grooming), or parts of them (such as grooming only the flank), which are performed out of context . When displacement activities become fixed and repetitive, they are described as stereotypies. In cats, these include repetitive vocalisation, running to and fro, polydypsia, polyphagia and chasing or staring at imaginary prey. The commonest stereotypy, however, is self-mutilation (Luescher *et al*, 1991) where a cat may groom its fur and cause baldness in certain areas or it may lick or chew itself, on occasion giving rise to tissue damage and chronic inflammation (see Chapter 9). When treating problems of this kind, care, of course, must also be taken to thoroughly investigate and treat any dermatological causes.

The mechanism and function of displacement activities and stereotypies are still unclear. It has been suggested (Dantzer, 1983) that they reduce tension and alleviate stress, perhaps because they generate endogenous endorphins. Although some stereotypies can be interrupted by the administration of naloxone, there is physiological evidence that stress is not reduced (Rushden, 1990). There may be a parallel between stereotypies in animals and obsessive compulsive disorders in humans. These patients report that although they carry out rituals such as repetitive hand-washing in order to reduce anxiety, their anxiety, in fact, tends to increase (Walker and Beech, 1968). It seems that a vicious circle may operate similar to that in which drug addicts are trapped.

# EARLY DEVELOPMENT

Chapter Five _____

Many owners know little or nothing about the early life of the cats they acquire. However, from the point of view of determining future behaviour, the first two months of life are critical for any cat.

## THE PERINATAL ENVIRONMENT

Most queens giving birth are left more to their own devices than are bitches, but not all are competent mothers and owners of breeding queens should be on hand to intervene if necessary. A primiparous mother, in particular, may be less efficient at cleaning the kittens after birth and, when cutting the umbilical cord with her teeth, may occasionally eat her kittens along with the placenta.

For the first three weeks of life, the kittens are entirely dependent on their mother for food and she initiates suckling. If she is under nourished during late pregnancy or during these early weeks, the behavioural development of the kittens tends to be adversely affected. Developmental milestones, such as eye opening, walking and playing will usually be delayed. Later in life, they show poorer learning ability and are likely to be more neurotic, showing higher levels of fear and aggression than kittens raised by adequately nourished mothers. (Smith & Jansen, 1977; Simonson, 1979). **This means that breeders must ensure adequate nutrition of breeding queens.** It is also an additional reason why kittens born to stray or feral mothers may not always make such good pets as those raised in a domestic setting (see page 31).

Although, by and large, breeders should not interfere unnecessarily with mother and kittens during the first weeks of life, it has been shown that, in common with other mammals such as rats and dogs, **some early handling is beneficial.** It tends to accelerate physical and behavioural development and to reduce fearfulness (Meier, 1961; Wilson, Warren and Abbott, 1965).

## TWO TO SEVEN WEEKS: THE SENSITIVE PERIOD

**The five weeks in a kitten's life after it first starts to hear, see and become mobile are critical for its future development.** Kittens separated from their mothers at two weeks old are likely to be more aggressive and nervous in later life (Seitz, 1959). Opportunity for social play with littermates is also critically important for a kitten's development. A kitten with no siblings will initiate play only with its mother and, although she usually responds, she does not spend as much time playing as littermates would. Whether this puts single kittens at disadvantage in later life is not yet known, but some single kittens, especially those raised by hand in isolation from other cats, are often hyper-reactive and, as adults, show a tendency to become aggressive when handled.

As well as playing a crucial role in her kittens' social and emotional development, the mother teaches them a range of more specific skills. Chesler (1969) found that kittens were able to learn a response of pressing a lever to obtain food only if they first observed their mother performing this task. Mothers probably also teach their kittens by demonstration to bury faeces and urine. They imitate her food preferences and maintain them even when she is absent. It seems likely, therefore, that a mother also has a strong influence on her kittens' attitude towards people: a friendly mother being more likely to have friendly kittens, for example, independent of any genetic effect.

A mother will also help her kittens to develop predatory skills by bringing them live, usually stunned, prey on which to practice prey handling and killing techniques. It is doubtful however, whether her experience and ability as a hunter affects her kittens' predatory skills with prey such as mice or small birds. These are relatively easy to kill: indeed, they are as likely to die from shock or clumsy handling by a kitten than from an accurate nape bite. Although experiments (Kuo, 1930) suggest that kittens tend to imitate their mother's choice of prey, it is doubtful whether this significantly influences the behaviour of most pet or feral cats: they tend to hunt the prey most abundant in their territory. However, prospective owners who are particularly concerned to minimise their cat's chances of catching birds might be advised to avoid the kittens of mothers who are enthusiastic bird hunters.

**The physical environment in which the kittens spend these first critical two months of life is also important.** Wilson et al (1965) found that kittens kept in a more complex, interesting environment were later less nervous when exploring a new situation than those raised in less stimulating surroundings. Ledger (1993) found that British Shorthair kittens reared by their breeders in isolated rooms were more fearful of a clockwork mouse and of a stranger than kittens reared in the midst of a normal domestic environment.

Most owners want a cat which is friendly and sociable towards themselves, their family and visitors. Although friendliness is probably genetically determined to some extent, it is also dependent on the kitten having adequate exposure to people during the first two months of life. Karsh has carried out a series of studies on this socialisation process (summarised by Karsh and Turner, 1988), demonstrating that its sensitive period lies between two and seven weeks of age. This period therefore theoretically comes to an end before weaning is completed naturally, normally at around eight weeks. Thus the responsibility for a kitten's social abilities with people rests predominantly with the breeder rather than with the new owner. This is another reason why the kittens of feral cats homed after 8 weeks of age often make unsatisfactory pets, despite efforts to socialise them later.

Karsh also found that the more contact kittens had with people during the sensitive period, the more sociable they tended to be in later life. Kittens which had contact with only one person did not generalise this friendliness to others, but kittens which had contact with at least four people were generally friendly with everyone they encountered. **Breeders should therefore spend as much time as possible with their kittens; they should also ensure that the kittens get to know at least a few other people as well.**

It used to be thought that this sensitive period for learning (which occurs in the young of most birds and social mammals) was strictly time-limited. It is now known that this differential learning capacity is not an "all or nothing" phenomenon. Learning opportunities missed during these first weeks of life can sometimes be made up later, although usually the process takes much longer.

Thus it is possible to socialise cats which have had no early exposure to people, but this is likely to need more time and patience than most ordinary pet owners are prepared to invest.

There is some evidence that such later socialisation can occur more quickly in adult life during periods of stress. Karsh recounts the case of a male laboratory cat, obtained as an adult, which she treated and nursed during a febrile illness. It thereafter followed her wherever possible. She suggests that this kind of process is mediated by noradrenalin facilitating neural plasticity. A similar explanation may apply to some accounts of feral cats captured as adults which become successful pets. Several similar cases have been encountered in practice of shy cats which had been friendly towards only one family member. Following periods of intensive nursing or confinement to a pen (for treatment for other behaviour problems) these cats became more generally friendly towards other members of the family and even friends.

There is also evidence (Bateson, 1987) that the part of the system which mediates learning of social attachments has a limited capacity and that different kinds of potential objects of attachment are in competition with one another. According to this model, biologically appropriate stimuli have preferential access to this system. For example, the results of experiments with a puppy reared with a litter of kittens (Kuo, 1960) confirm this. If any of the kittens was separated from the rest of the litter, it cried: this crying was reduced by the presence of any one of the rest of the litter, including the puppy. However, the presence of any of the other kittens reduced the crying more than the presence of the puppy. People stand in the same relation to a litter of kittens as the puppy in Kuo's experiment, in that we are in competition for their social attachment with the biologically advantageous mother and littermates. This further emphasises the need for breeders to spend as much time as possible with their kittens in order to maximise the chances of their being as friendly towards people as they are towards other cats.

It is worth bearing in mind, however, that early handling does not ensure the development of a friendly disposition in a kitten, presumably because of genetic or other constitutional factors. Karsh found that even under the best experimental conditions about 15% of her kittens seemed to resist socialisation. On the other hand, it is possible that a remedial regime designed for these kittens might have been effective. **Some responsible breeders observe their kittens closely and give individual attention to shy or fearful kittens: all breeders should be encouraged to do this.**

## FURTHER READING

TURNER D. C. and BATESON P. (Eds). (1988). The Human-Cat Relationship. In *The Domestic Cat The Biology of Its Behaviour*. Cambridge University Press. Chapters 2,3,4 and 12.

# OWNER ATTITUDES

Chapter Six ─────────────────────────────────

**Veterinary surgeons may assume that cat owners are on the whole less attached to their pets than dog owners. The evidence on this point is conflicting**. Wilbur (1976), carrying out a cluster analysis of attitude questionnaire responses by dog and cat owners, found three categories of cat owners: high involvement owners, who relied on their cats for love and affection (20%); quality/status conscious owners who were more concerned with the image that their cat and the rest of their domestic situation presented to the world (21%); and low involvement owners who had no great affection for their cat, but chose it as a pet because it required little care and attention (59%). Dog owners fell into five categories: companion owners (27%) who regarded their dogs as members of the family; enthusiastic owners (17%) who enjoyed their dogs but were less involved with them; worried owners (24%) who were attached to their dogs but were upset or embarrassed by their behaviour; valued object owners (19%) who seemed to have no emotional tie with their dog but viewed them as possessions, and dissatisfied owners (19%) who derived no satisfaction from their dogs and felt them to be a nuisance. Setting aside the one-fifth of dog and cat owners who are valued object/status conscious owners, this seems to leave 68% of dog owners emotionally attached to their dogs, compared with 20% of cat owners.

On the other hand, a survey by Voith (1985) found that 99% of both dog and cat owners considered their pets to be family members. In each case, 97% talked to their pet at least once a day and 91% had photographs of them. However, as pointed out in Chapter 1, Voith's sample was self-selected and was therefore probably biased towards highly attached owners. Catanzaro (1988) surveyed 961 pet-owning clients attending US Army Veterinary Corps clinics. He found that only 68% of these clients considered their pets to be family members. **It seems likely that both the absolute proportion of cat owners who are highly attached to their pets and the proportion relative to dog owners varies according to the population under survey.** So far, there is little evidence on the kind of people who are likely to be more attached to their cats, but it seems probable that the factors which dispose to high attachment are similar to those known to apply to dog owners (O'Farrell, 1992) i.e. being single or childless or being in need of emotional support. In addition, animals which have been hand reared are often felt to be special, as are pets inherited from dead relatives.

Cultural factors also influence the strength of the attachments which owners allow themselves to form with their pets. In nineteenth century Britain, it was generally accepted that civilized man should dominate and exploit other animal species, as well as other people in under developed countries. Those who responded to this authoritarian attitude with submission, devotion and loyalty (e.g. dogs, Ghurkas) were rewarded with affection and approval. Those who persisted in maintaining their independence (e.g. cats, "savages") were hated and feared (Ritvo, 1985). Since then, attitudes have gradually changed and it is now more generally accepted that the behaviour patterns and ways of life of other species should be respected. The increase in popularity of the cat may be linked to this change in attitude. However as Serpell (1988) points out, the idea still persists that, among men, cat ownership is often associated with homosexuality i.e. "real men don't keep cats".

With this kind of attitude still prevalent, the veterinary surgeon should bear in mind that **owners may conceal the strength of their attachment to their cats**. Catanzaro found that, over a range of measures, the veterinarians in his study substantially underestimated the degree of their clients' attachment to their pets . Although an owner who is emotionally dependent on his or her cat may make the veterinary surgeon feel uncomfortable, strong attachment on the part of the owner is a good prognostic factor in the treatment of behaviour problems. The treatment of these problems requires time, patience and disruption of domestic routine for the owners. Those who are not very attached to their cats in the first place may simply not be prepared to take the necessary trouble. However, as with physical treatment, it is sometimes possible to devise less demanding regimes which produce sufficient improvement to make the cat's behaviour more acceptable to the owner. Alternatively, a treatment plan unveiled in instalments may be less daunting for these owners.

As well as the intensity of the cat/owner relationship, its nature is also relevant. It is a commonly held view that many emotionally attached owners treat their cats or dogs as children. There is now evidence to support this. For example Voith, (1985), in her survey of owners of 800 cats, found that 59% said that they talked to their cat "as a child" at least sometimes, and 37% talked to it as a child all the time. Berryman et al (1985), administered a Kelly Repertory Grid (a psychological test designed to reveal how a subject views the world, using his own concepts) to 30 owners of pets, comprising mostly cats and dogs. They found that most of the owners saw their relationship with their pet as most similar to a relationship with a child.

However, a view of a pet as child is an over-simplification. In only one instance of eight Repertory Grids administered to dog owners (O'Farrell, 1994) was the subject's favourite dog seen as closest to "child". For six subjects the relationship was seen as being closest to "mother". Of course, the owners involved in such studies are aware that their pets are not really people. In describing a cat or dog as being "like a child" or "like a mother", they are stating how it fulfils particular needs for them. If a pet is seen as "like a child", this may mean that it satisfies an owner's need to look after someone. If it is "like a parent", the owner may feel that the pet protects him or her. Although dogs have a more obvious protective function, 33% of the owners in Voith's survey also felt protected by their cats, mostly because they alerted them to strange noises.

Additionally, both dogs and cats may be seen by their owners as close friends or confidants. In Voith's study, more cat owners (58%) than dog owners (45%) said that they talked to their pet about important matters at least once a month. On the other hand, 99% of dog owners, as opposed to 89% of cat owners, believed they were aware of their pet's moods, and 98% of dog owners, as opposed to 91% of cat owners, believed that their pet was aware of their own moods.

The clientele of almost every veterinary practice usually includes at least one person concerned with cat rescue or welfare work. Many of these owners end up keeping more cats than most people would consider tolerable. Most derive obvious satisfaction from their cat family and many simply cannot bear to turn away any cat. Some may eventually be unable to cope with the burden of numbers they have taken on and may have to be tactfully rescued from their rescuing. As might be expected, problems such as aggression and territorial marking tend to increase with the number of cats in the household (see pages 47 and 60). At a certain critical density of cat population, however, these problems seem to decrease: over crowding seems to have an inhibiting effect on many such social interactions.

One important practical question which arises from these considerations is which kinds of cat/owner relationship are most likely to be satisfactory to both cat and owner. Little work has been done in this area. However, psychoanalysts working with intimate human/human relationships, such as marriage, have pointed out that difficulties are more likely to arise when partners fail to regard each other as separate individuals with their own personalities but instead project their own needs onto the other partner (Scharff & Scharff, 1991). The higher a person's general levels of anxiety and conflict (i.e., the more neurotic he or she is), the greater will be his or her need to engage in projection of this kind.

Similar processes may occur in human/dog relationships (O'Farrell, 1992, 1994). Sometimes, for example, it is evident that a behavioural problem is being aggravated by the owner's unrealistic or self-contradictory expectations, based on his own needs or anxieties. Dogs may also be idealised: a study using the Kelly Repertory Grid found that idealisation was most common in owners who, as children, had had an unsatisfactory relationship with their same sex parent (O'Farrell, 1994).

Whether the same processes occur in cat/owner relationships is open to question. Certainly, on occasion, **an owner's own needs can give rise to unrealistic expectations of his cat, which in turn can cause problems.**

## Case History 1

*Miss S., a journalist in her forties, sought help because Sammy, a six-year-old domestic short-haired male neuter, had started to defaecate away from the litter tray. Miss S. lived in a flat of which two rooms were let out to lodgers. She had two other cats, both male neuters aged eight and four, but there was no animosity between any of the cats and they regularly played together. Miss S. professed herself completely devoted to her cats, which, for no clear reason, were allowed outside only for short periods, under supervision. During the day, the cats had access to Miss S.'s bed/sitting room, the kitchen and hallway. She excluded them from her bedroom at night, because they tried to play with her and disturbed her sleep. Though there were litter trays in hallway and kitchen, the misplaced defaecation usually occurred on the kitchen table and at night. The lodgers, though generally tolerant, had begun to complain.*

*It emerged during the interview that Miss S. had recently acquired her first dog: a four-month-old German Shepherd from an animal shelter. It seemed that the dog, though quite difficult to handle, showed no aggression towards the cats, which kept out of its way as best they could. The dog was also excluded from Miss S.'s bedroom at night because he took up too much room in the bed.*

*Miss S.'s morning routine was to get up, visit the bathroom and then make herself a cup of coffee in the kitchen. After that, she retired to her room to dress, which took about ten minutes. It was during these ten minutes that Sammy was most likely to defaecate on the table.*

*When it was suggested to Miss S. that the addition of the dog to her household had been stressful to the cats, particularly to Sammy, her reaction was guarded. It seemed likely that friends or the referring veterinary surgeon had already pointed this out, but that she had been unwilling to accept the implications. It was further suggested that Sammy was most likely to defaecate on the table in the mornings because the cats and dog, having been aroused by Miss S.'s appearance in the kitchen, were then left alone together when she withdrew to her room. Sammy was probably deterred from using one of the litter trays by the fact that the dog had access to both of them and could disturb him. When this was pointed out, Miss S. became rather defensive. She was not willing to modify her morning routine in the slightest particular: for example, by dressing before she left the bedroom or by taking the dog into the bedroom with her while she dressed. Other therapeutic suggestions based on a change of routine met with similar objections.*

*It seemed that Miss S. needed the company of her cats (and now her dog) to such an extent that she could not contemplate parting with any of them. But the attachment seemed to blind her to the fact that the animals' needs and emotions could be different from her own. She could not, for example, appreciate that they might not all enjoy one another's company as much as she enjoyed theirs; nor that they might need her presence when she did not want theirs.*

The case of Miss S. is not uncommon. Many pet owners have not considered what effect they or their lifestyle is having on their cat. Explaining what, to the veterinary surgeon, may seem the simple or obvious needs of a pet may require great patience and take up a large proportion of some behaviour consultations.

There is also evidence that, on a more subtle level, subjugation of the cat's emotional needs to those of the owner tends to result in a less satisfactory relationship. Turner and Stammbach-Geering (1990, 1991) studied 158 Swiss housewives and their cats, observing their interactions over three days. The owners were asked to rate their cats and their "ideal" cats on a range of characteristics. They also assessed their own attitudes towards the real and ideal cat.

Studying the pattern of interactions between cat and owner, Turner found a statistically significant correlation (.32) between the owner's willingness to comply with the cat's wish to interact and the cat's willingness to comply with the owner's wish to interact. In other words, the more the owner responds to the cat, the more likely the cat is to respond to the owner. As already mentioned (page 22), for a given cat/owner pair, the more interactions initiated by the cat, the longer these interactions lasted. Although this correlation was fairly low (only accounting for 10% of the total variance), it is important because it highlights a difference between dog/owner and cat/owner relationships. Dogs of most breeds and types instinctively expect to live in a dominance hierarchy and, in that hierarchy, dominant individuals will tend to initiate rather than respond to social interactions. For a dog that is inclined to be dominant in the human pack, the more its owner complies with its wishes, the more likely it is that the dog will perceive him or her as a subordinate and the less likely it is, therefore, to comply with its owner's wishes.

Although about a quarter of dog and cat owners keep both species (Beta Petfoods, 1991), many conform to the popular stereotypes of either being dog owners who dislike cats or cat owners who dislike dogs. It also seems likely that some of the dog owners conform even further to the first stereotype and are authoritarian and controlling people who dislike the cat's "independence". Interestingly, when Adorno *et al* (1950) developed the concept of the authoritarian personality in people and devised a questionnaire (the F scale) to measure it, they found that agreement with the statement "dogs are much more admirable animals than cats" was as highly correlated with "authoritarianism" as any other item in the questionnaire.

Certainly **some dog owners seem to derive their main satisfaction of ownership from controlling their dogs and giving them commands. A cat owner who looks for this kind of satisfaction is doomed to disappointment.** Further results from Turner and Stammbach-Geering's study seem to confirm this. They found, not surprisingly, that owners tended to prefer cats which are affectionate, playful, predictable and which display curiosity. They also liked cats which were clean and used the litter tray but not cats which sprayed urine or which were active at night. The study also found that owners who were more willing to respond to their cat's desire to interact (a recipe for a successful relationship) tended to perceive both their real and their ideal cat as being more independent in character. Not surprisingly, they were more likely to be owners of cats which were allowed access to the outdoors. Indoor cats tend to have more behaviour problems than cats which have access to outdoors (Neville, 1992). This may be because outdoor cats can go out to engage in behaviour such as territorial marking which is unacceptable indoors; or it may be because their owners cannot manage undesirable behaviour by shutting the cat out. However, it may also be because owners of indoor cats tend to try to exert more control over the relationship than is good for it and thus are more likely to become dissatisfied when it fails to match their expectations.

In the case of dogs, unrealistic needs of the owner can lead to problems not only because the dog falls short of expectations but because, in some cases, the owner's anxiety itself may raise the dog's own level of stress. Dogs owned by neurotic owners tend themselves to exhibit more neurotic behaviour in the form of overexcitement and stereotypies (O'Farrell, 1992). This may be because anxious owners tend to pay more attention to peculiar behaviour, such as a stereotypy, or annoying behaviour, such as overexcitement. Because for most dogs, the owner's attention acts as a powerful reward, such behaviours will be reinforced and thus tend to show a proportionate increase. In addition, an anxious owner may behave more inconsistently towards his dog, unpredictably rewarding and punishing the same behaviour, producing a state of conflict in the dog and leading to stress related behaviour changes (see Chapter 4). Although most cats tend to be less motivated than dogs by the desire for their owner's attention, the same mechanism can sometimes be seen in operation, particularly in very sociable cats. For example, excessive grooming may start, or may recur at times of crisis in the family.

On the whole, however, it may well be that cats are less affected by the emotional distress of their owners. Cats, or at least the more independent minded individuals, might therefore be recommended as suitable pets for certain types of owner with anxiety problems, though this area warrants further investigation.

The veterinary surgeon should also bear in mind that some people fear or hate cats. Those who feel the same way about dogs often use a legitimate concern, such as fear of attack or fouling in public places, as a vehicle for their irrational emotions, but prejudice against cats is, on the whole, more nakedly expressed. Cat haters may often refer to the same characteristics of independence and unpredictability which mar the enjoyment for some cat owners, although, for other owners, it is these same characteristics which make the cat so attractive and fascinating.

There is little information on fear of cats but research has thrown some light on hatred of cats when expressed as cruelty. Although the Scottish Society for the Prevention of Cruelty to Animals is responsible for eight times as many successful prosecutions involving dogs than those involving cats, the proportion of the cases involving violence (rather than neglect or abandonment) is twice as high for cats as for dogs (Watt, 1991). Felthous (1981), interviewing 346 male psychiatric patients found that, of the 18 subjects who had repeatedly tortured cats or dogs, 17 had tortured cats, nearly three times as many as had tortured dogs. In another study involving prisoners, Kellert and Felthous (1985) found that subjects reported inflicting more severe forms of cruelty on cats than on dogs (e.g. exploding them in a microwave oven or shooting them for target practice, as compared with beating them or entering them in dog fights). Cruelty to the dogs was often used as a form of severe discipline or in order to enhance the subject's self-esteem, even though the subjects often professed affection for their dogs. In contrast, the cats were frequently abused because they were hated and were described as "sneaky", "creepy", "treacherous" or "spooky". People who are afraid of cats often use similar terms to describe the aspects of the cat which they find alarming.

In western culture, there is a strong historical precedent for prejudice against cats. In ancient Egypt and in pre-Christian Europe they were seen as benevolent symbols of femininity and associated with mother goddesses such as Minerva, Diana and Freya. With the spread of Christianity and the eradication of pagan beliefs, they came to be associated with heresy and devil worship; society condoned their persecution and torture. As late as the nineteenth century, cats were regarded as the archetypal witches' familiar (Serpell, 1988).

There seems little doubt that this loathing of cats was linked to the Christian church's ambivalence towards, and its condemnation and fear of, female sexuality. As Serpell points out, the cat's appearance and behaviour have made it a symbol of a negative perception of women: beautiful, graceful and soft to the touch, but inscrutable and unpredictable in their social interactions. The association with female sexuality still persists in the use of slang terms, such as "pussy", for the female genitalia.

Prejudice against cats may now be diminishing. However, there is evidence that it persists to some extent even in professions which are in a position to advise cat owners. In a questionnaire completed by 206 American physicians specialising in the treatment of allergy (Bates and McCulloch, 1983), 83% considered cats to be the animal species most likely to cause allergy: 34% said they would recommend removal of the pet even if the patient was not exhibiting allergic symptoms to it. Those who themselves owned or had owned a pet were significantly less likely to make this recommendation.

In a study of the attitudes of veterinary students (O'Farrell, unpublished data), 34 third year students were asked to rate a dog and a cat of their acquaintance on various scales such as loving, playful etc. Dogs were rated as significantly more loving, interesting, reliable, playful and sensitive to the owner's moods, though they were also rated as more annoying. Veterinary surgeons themselves should therefore guard against a prejudice against cats, which might lead them, for example, to underestimate clients' attachment to their cats.

# DIAGNOSIS AND TREATMENT OF BEHAVIOUR PROBLEMS

Chapter Seven _____

## DIAGNOSIS

The diagnosis of behaviour problems requires a different approach to the diagnosis of most physical problems. Although it may be helpful to find a label for the cat's problem behaviour (e.g. urine marking, redirected aggression) this label does not normally on its own provide adequate information on which to base a treatment regime. Most problems are caused by a unique combination of multiple factors. An explanation of the behaviour in terms of these factors must be formulated before treatment can be planned.

Physical causes may, of course, play a part in some behavioural problems. For example, urination in the house may be associated with the onset of a urinary tract infection. Although it is essential to diagnose and treat any such physical problems, diagnoses of physical and behavioural disorders should not be regarded as mutually exclusive. For instance, although a cat may sometimes be forced to urinate in the house because of urgency and frequency caused by an infection, the behaviour may become classically conditioned and so continue long after the infection has been successfully treated. The more chronic the physical disorder, the more likely it is to acquire behavioural components. For example, a cat may aggravate a dermatological disorder by excessive licking and over-grooming and such problems may need, from the outset, to be treated with a combination of physical and behavioural approaches.

### Taking a history

It is impossible to arrive at the correct explanation of a behavioural problem without first eliciting adequate information from the owner. The cat's behaviour should also be observed, including, if possible, the problem behaviour. More time must be allocated for this than would normally be spent on a routine veterinary consultation.

The information elicited should include answers to the following questions:

### What exactly is the problem? What does the cat do?
General descriptive terms are not sufficient. "Nervous", for example, may mean fearful, excitable or even aggressive. Detailed information about the cat's body posture may also be important, for instance, when distinguishing between different types of urination or aggression: owners may need help in describing accurately their pet's body language and vocalisations. Unfortunately,

only a small proportion of problematic behaviours can be elicited in the surgery: where possible, video film taken by the owner can be a useful adjunct to consultation. If the owner's description is unclear or incomplete, a home visit may be necessary for first hand observations of the cat and its lifestyle.

**In which situations does the problem behaviour occur?** Successful treatment often depends on defining the trigger of the behaviour in detail. **Which people or other animals are normally present? What are they usually doing before, during and after the behaviour occurs? Where does the behaviour occur?** The layout of the house and sometimes of the garden is often important. If the consultation takes place away from the owner's house, she should be encouraged to draw a map showing relevant features such doors, cat flaps, dogs' or cats' beds, litter trays etc.

**When and under what circumstances did the problem first occur?** It should be borne in mind, however, that a problem which started for one reason may persist for another. For example, urine spraying triggered by a single territorial invasion by another cat may be maintained long afterwards by classical conditioning.

**What treatment methods, if any, are the owners trying or have they already tried?** It is often necessary to obtain a detailed description of these. Some methods, punishment for example, may be making the problem worse. Other methods, such as effective cleaning of urine marks, may be helping to contain the problem. Others may have failed not because the general method was inappropriate but because some of the details need refinement or modification. Thus, systematic desensitization may fail if it proceeds at too fast a rate. In these cases, the practitioner needs only to advise the client how to modify the treatment rather than to design a completely new regime.

It is vital to learn as much as possible about the cat's general behaviour and character. For example, if it is suffering from a specific phobia, it is important to determine whether it is generally fearful, excitable or placid by nature: on this may depend the nature and pace of treatment. It may also determine whether drug support is likely to be helpful. **Is the cat currently undergoing any form of medical treatment involving stressful handling, change of lifestyle or drug therapy? Are there other behaviour problems?** Clients may not initially present the problem which bothers them most, especially if describing the main problem causes them embarrassment, for example if they are houseproud and their cat defaecates indoors.

**What is the cat's daily routine? Is it an indoor cat or does it have free or limited access to outdoors?** If so, how much time does it spend away from home and what does it do? When at home, where does it eat and sleep? How much time do owner and cat spend interacting? What do they do together? Is there gentle petting and cuddling and do they play together? What form does the play take: does it involve manipulating objects for the cat to stalk and pounce on or does it involve physical rough-and-tumble?

**What is the composition of the household? Are there other cats or dogs? What are the behaviour and attitudes of the rest of the family towards the cat?** The aggressive or excitable behaviour of a new puppy or the hostile and punitive attitude of a human family member may be a source of stress. The views and attitude of family members toward the problem are also relevant. It is important that misconceptions (for example, that the cat is acting out of spite) be revealed, in order that these may be corrected. Also, the clinician should find out how close the owners are to wishing to rid themselves of the cat. This has a direct bearing on treatment. It may, for example, determine whether a behaviour therapy regime should be supplemented with drugs. Even if the effect of the drug is only temporary it may encourage the owner to continue with treatment.

## Formulating An Explanation

To arrive at an accurate diagnosis, the following framework may be helpful:

### Interpretation of the behaviour

It is important to identify the instinctive behavioural sequence of which the problem behaviour is a part. This is most likely to be determined from observation, from exact description of the cat's behaviour or from identification of the triggering stimuli. In addition, does the behaviour show stereotypic features (see page 54)? Is there a learned component to the behaviour? This should be suspected if the behaviour is regularly followed by a rewarding event, such as the owner's attention. It should also be suspected if a triggering stimulus has generalised from that which originally provoked the behaviour to other stimuli: if, for example, territorial aggression towards an intruding cat has generalised to aggression towards another resident cat.

### Causative factors

As explained above, a behaviour problem is likely to be the result of a combination of causative factors. A hormonal influence should be suspected if the behaviour is dimorphic such as urine spraying by intact male cats and inter-male aggression. Synthetic progestagens or anti-androgens are likely to be most helpful in such cases, occasionally in isolation, but more often as adjuncts to behaviour therapy.

Genetic factors are likely to be involved in problems which are more common in particular breeds, for example fabric eating in Siamese cats. If the problem has been present since the cat was a kitten, genetic or constitutional factors or disruptions in the early environment are likely to be involved. In these cases, modification of the behaviour or its redirection onto a less problematic target, rather than complete disappearance of the behaviour, is a realistic goal of treatment.

Anxiety or stress is likely to be a causative factor if the cat has become more fearful and withdrawn or more excitable and easily aroused. This should also be suspected if the onset of the problem has coincided with a potentially stressful event, such as separation from the owner, addition or loss of a human or animal member to the household or the arrival of a new cat or dog in the immediate neighbourhood.

The clinician should also reflect on whether the owner's attitude towards the cat might be contributing to the problem. For instance, the owner might be overestimating the cat's cognitive abilities or have an inappropriately moralistic attitude (see chapter 2) or his emotional dependence might be leading him to curtail the cat's freedom of movement in a way which places undue stress upon it (see case history page 35).

## TREATMENT

This section outlines the treatment options available to the clinician. These should not be viewed as mutually exclusive.

### Surgical Treatment

In cats, it is universally accepted that the benefits of castration outweigh the risks and this operation is performed routinely on most male pet cats. There is evidence (Hart & Barrett, 1973) that castration of adult tom cats eliminates or markedly reduces spraying and fighting in 90% of cases. There is also evidence (Hart & Cooper, 1984) that a similar percentage of male cats castrated before puberty will similarly benefit. These authors suggest that these findings taken together imply that pre- and post-pubertal castration are equally effective in eliminating spraying.

The evidence is not so clear with regard to the effects of castration on inter-male fighting. But, in any case, pre-pubertal castration is usually advisable, both for population control and its beneficial effects on other behaviours such as roaming.

Other surgical treatments for spraying have been proposed, such as olfactory tractotomy (Hart, 1982) and bilateral ischiocavaernosus myectomy (Komtebedde & Hauptman, 1990). These techniques must be regarded at present as experimental. As a treatment for territorial scratching, declawing is much less popular in Great Britain than in North America. Presumably this is partly due to the fact that a higher proportion of British cats go outdoors. There is evidence, however, (Landsberg, 1991) that most outdoor cats are not handicapped by declawing. On the other hand, territorial scratching is less likely than spraying to be an intolerable problem to most owners. All of these surgical interventions (olfactory tractotomy, ischiocavaernosus myectomy and declawing) must significantly interfere with the cat's quality of life. Although in theory there might be cases where they are the only alternatives to euthanasia, other treatment methods or rehoming are almost always preferable and more appropriate.

The surgical treatment of a stereotypy by removal of one of the body parts involved (e.g. treatment of tail chasing by removing the tail) is absolutely contra-indicated. Such an approach is hardly ever successful and the discomfort produced by the wound may well aggravate the problem.

Any surgical treatment should be immediately followed by behavioural treatment in order to maximise its effect by dealing with factors such as learning or environmental stress not addressed by the surgery.

## Drug Treatment

As with surgery, drug treatment should always be accompanied by behavioural treatment and preceded by a thorough clinical examination. The risk of adverse effects must be weighed against possible benefits. The fact that a drug has been licensed for animal use does not necessarily imply the most favourable balance of risks and benefits. Veterinary surgeons who prescribe unlicensed drugs however, should be particularly careful to warn clients to watch out for adverse side effects, especially in the first few days of their administration. Some anxiolytics, such as diazepam, inhibit learning. They should therefore be prescribed carefully and in tapered doses, especially when administered in conjunction with regimes such as systematic desensitization. The doses advised below have been derived from current literature and care should be taken to note that some drug dosages are given **per cat and not per kilogram**.

The peak of the popularity of progestagens has probably passed. Of these the most widely used in behavioural treatment is megestrol acetate (Ovarid, Pitman-Moore). Its anti-androgenic effects reduce urine spraying (see page 62) and inter-male aggression (see pages 46-47). Because of its limbic effects (as yet poorly understood), it can also be helpful in the treatment of stress-related disorders, especially those resulting from a single traumatic event, such as the loss of a close companion, a change of house or an attack by another cat. It is less likely to be effective for a problem arising from ongoing social pressures, such as poor relations with another cat in the household. Doses of 2.5-5mg/cat daily for seven days, then 2.5-5mg/cat weekly have been recommended (Marder, 1991). Treatment with progestagens is not without risk however: adverse metabolic and endocrinological effects can occur without external signs (Henik et al, 1985) and their probability increases with length of use. It is therefore desirable to give the lowest possible therapeutic dose and a dose which is half the recommended dose may be effective in some cats.

In contrast, the popularity of the benzodiazepines (e.g. diazepam (Valium, Roche)) has increased as evidence has emerged that they can provide a safer and effective treatment, not only for disorders such as phobias, but also for problems such as urine spraying (see page 62) and aggression (see page 47). The recommended dose of diazepam is 1-2mg/cat b.i.d. (Voith, 1989) although doses as high as 5mg/cat t.i.d. have been used without ill effect (Hart & Hart, 1985). Cats show a wide variation in sensitivity to this drug and it occasionally provokes a paradoxical reaction of excitement and over-activity. It is therefore usually advisable to administer a low dose initially: if this is ineffective, the dose should be increased rapidly to avoid habituation. If the cat's level of activity is markedly suppressed or if it becomes ataxic, the dose should be reduced. Some cats are so sensitive to the drug that it is impossible to find a dose which reduces anxiety without unacceptable sedation.

More recently, the tricyclic antidepressants have been successfully used to reduce anxiety. The most frequently employed is amitriptyline at a dosage for cats of 0.5-1mg/kg. A combination of phenobarbitone (1-2mg/kg b.i.d.) and propranalol (1-2mg/kg b.i.d.) has also been found to be effective in reducing anxiety (Walker, personal communication). Contraindications include use in animals with bradycardia, hypotension or heart failure.

Recently, long-acting opioid antagonists such as naltrexone (Nalorex, DuPont) have been found useful in the treatment of stereotypies (see page 54) at a dose of 2.5-5mg/cat for seven days then 2.5-5mg/cat weekly.

## Behavioural Treatment

In planning a regime for behavioural treatment, the following framework may be useful:

### Stress reduction
Where there is evidence that the cat is stressed, the source of stress should, if possible, be eliminated. If, for example, other cats are invading the house, they might be excluded by blocking up the cat flap. Alternatively, it might be replaced with a selective model which, by means of a magnetic or electronic "key" worn on the collar, allows access only to the resident cat. If the source of stress cannot be removed (for example, if the other cats live in the same household) the cat should be provided with a safe haven where it can escape from the stress. If neither of these alternatives is feasible, it may be necessary to provide drug support to help the cat adapt to the stress or cope with the behaviour of the other cats.

### Redirecting instinctive behaviour
Where instinctive behaviour is involved, some attempt may be made to redirect it on to a more acceptable object. For instance, if the owner is the victim of predatory assaults, she might divert the attacks onto moving toys which she carries with her around the house for use as required.

### Rearrangement of rewards
Where it is suspected that the behaviour has been acquired via instrumental learning and is maintained by rewards, the timings of these rewards should, if possible, be altered so that acceptable rather than unacceptable behaviour is reinforced. Thus, if it seems that a cat's constant mewing is being rewarded by the owner's attention, the owner should ignore the cat when it mews, but pay it attention when it is quiet.

### Systematic desensitization
When an emotion, such as fear, aggression or excitement, has been conditioned to an undesirable stimulus, it should be treated by systematic desensitization as described on page 27.

### Modifying owner attitudes
Where the owners attitude towards or relationship with the cat seems to be a factor in maintaining the problem behaviour or in preventing its treatment, some attempt must be made to modify it. Obviously, this is an area which must be approached with tact. Judgmental statements should be avoided and, where possible, concrete, practical suggestions made. The owners may need time

and discussion in order to absorb what may be, for them, new and threatening ideas. It is often appropriate for the veterinary surgeon to indicate that the owners' feelings or attitudes are natural and understandable. For example, if the clinician suspects that an owner's moralistic and punitive attitude towards his cat is a factor in maintaining its spraying behaviour, he might sympathise with the anger, but suggest that a specific expression of it - namely, punishing the cat - is making matters worse.

## WHEN TREATMENT FAILS

Inevitably, in some cases, treatment fails or is not even feasible to embark on. For some dogs, the decision as to what to do next is fairly clear: some dogs pose such an immediate threat to people that euthanasia is the only option and the veterinary surgeon has little hesitation in recommending it, even if there is a possibility that treatment might reduce the risk of injury. Few cats, however, fall into this category, although some may be an intolerable danger to other cats in the household. A problem cat is more likely to be rehomed or euthanased because the owner is no longer prepared to tolerate its behaviour. The tolerance of owners varies enormously. Although some are prepared to live with a level of dirt or destruction which the clinician would not find acceptable personally, others appear to set impossibly high standards for their cat's behaviour. In such cases, the veterinary surgeon may be called upon to destroy what seems to be a normal cat. Although cat rescue societies may sometimes be able to help, new homes for unwanted cats can be hard to find and the veterinary surgeon may have to accept this unpleasant role as philosophically as he can.

In some cases, a behaviour problem may disappear completely if a cat is rehomed. This sometimes applies, for instance, to a cat which is showing aggression towards other cats in the household. Again, such cats may have to be destroyed simply because no new home can be found.

Equally distressing for the clinician are the cases which seem treatable, but whose owners are unwilling to embark on treatment. Finding a successful treatment regime often requires time and patience. Even more difficult for the clinician can be the clients who are willing to try treatment but who make it clear that their patience will soon be exhausted. For these cats, the knowledge that it may be a matter of life or death whether the correct treatment is found sooner rather than later subjects the veterinary surgeon to extra pressure.

## FURTHER READING

MARDER, A. R. (1991). Psychotropic drugs and behavioural therapy. *Veterinary Clinics of North America* **21**, 329-342

# PROBLEMS OF AGGRESSION

Chapter Eight

Before trying to treat a problem of aggression in a cat, it is important first to identify it correctly. The contexts in which it occurs, when it first occurred and the cat's body postures and vocalisations at the time are crucial. The cat's age and sex are also relevant, as are the characteristics of the victims including, if they are cats, their age and sex. It should be borne in mind, however, that what started out as one type of aggression can, over time, change into another.

## PREDATORY BEHAVIOUR

Predatory behaviour differs from other forms of aggression in that it tends to be silent and consists of sequences of behaviour, such as stalk, pounce, grasp, bite etc., which are not found in the same sequence or expressed in the same manner as in social encounters with other cats or people. In such social encounters, aggression is part of a system of communication between the two parties involved. When hunting, the object is not to communicate with the prey, but simply to capture, kill and eat it.

If they have the opportunity, most cats will hunt and kill small animals such as birds and mice, although some are more enthusiastic and skilful hunters than others. Although most owners are philosophical and learn to live with this aspect of a cat's instinctive behavioural repertoire, some are upset by it. It may be some comfort to them to reflect that cats evolved into predators over millions of years, long before they were domesticated.

Certainly owners should not be encouraged to believe that they can abolish their cats' hunting behaviour, although they might be able to reduce its effectiveness. Cats are predominantly crepuscular hunters: keeping them indoors at dawn and dusk, when rodents tend to be active, may reduce the carnage to some extent. Protecting fledglings during the nesting season of garden birds may prove more difficult. Feeding a cat before favourite hunting times may reduce its eagerness a little. Feeding fresh gristly meat still attached to the bone may increase the effect somewhat, although a full stomach probably reduces the number of animals killed because it makes the cat sleepy or slower, rather than because it directly affects the cat's motivation to hunt. Attaching a bell to the cat's collar may allow more alert and agile victims to escape. It is usually best, however, to encourage clients to tolerate and manage this aspect of their cats' behaviour, rather than trying to alter it. Owners may be less upset by their cat's hunting if it does not bring the results into the house. They may be able to deter the cat from doing this by hissing at it when it comes indoors with its prey. They may simply bar entry by keeping doors shut and dispensing with or locking the cat flap.

## PLAY AGGRESSION

Play aggression may contain components of intra-species aggression, but often most closely resembles predatory behaviour. It differs from it in that the components may appear jumbled up and out of sequence and the attack is, to some extent, inhibited. Thus the victim may be stalked and pounced on but not "killed," the force of the bite being reduced and claws retracted. However, as with true predatory behaviour, the attacks are seldom accompanied by any vocalisation.

Cats may play with toys and with each other; they may also show play aggression towards their owners. Borchelt & Voith (1987) have found play aggression to be the most common form of aggression directed at people. Although this type of aggression is most common in kittens and young cats, mature cats may continue to try to play in this way. Owners may find this alarming, especially if they do not understand their cat's behaviour. Even an inhibited attack can cause some injury, particularly to young children, the elderly or the infirm.

Such attacks are almost always triggered by movement of the victim. The cat may lie in wait, perhaps in a favourite place, to ambush people as they go by. He may also have a favourite victim/playmate target. **Owners should not try to deter the cat from this behaviour by counter-attacking** with attempts to strike it or push it away. There is a danger that, even if the cat is not alarmed by these actions, it may interpret them as reciprocal play. If it is alarmed, it may show defensive aggression, thus making the problem worse.

Confining or isolating the cat is unlikely to improve matters. **Playful cats need to be played with**. Inexperienced owners may need advice on suitable toys and how to move them erratically in order to elicit and sustain play behaviour. Owners of these cats should be encouraged to play with them more frequently. More specifically, they should use toys to deflect attacks directed towards themselves. The more accurately the time and place of these attacks can be predicted, the greater is the chance that they can be prevented. Owners might, for example, throw a toy ahead of them as they pass the cat's favourite spot for an ambush. They might also throw a toy to divert the cat's attention if it becomes overexcited.

## INTER-MALE AGGRESSION

Typically entire tom cats engage in instinctive competitive behaviour. However, Hart (Hart and Cooper, 1984; Hart and Barrett, 1973) has found that 44% of castrated male cats fight with other cats at least occasionally and 10% engage in serious fighting. The proportions engaging in inter-male aggression must be less than these, however, as the same study found that 30% of female cats also fight at least occasionally.

Inter-male aggression can normally be distinguished from other types of fighting by the characteristic threat ritual which precedes it. Typically the aggressor assumes a confident stance. The tail may be held stiffly up, turning down at the end and twitching. The ears face forward and the head may be slightly tilted from side to side. There is usually a good deal of growling, spitting and miaowing. This threat ritual may last for some time, with the cats moving slowly towards or away from each other. The fight, if it occurs, though often dramatic and accompanied by screaming, is usually comparatively brief. There may be several rounds of threat and fight before the encounter is over. The fights seldom result in serious injuries, except when the back feet are employed to rake at the stomach of the opponent. More often, the chief danger to the fighting cat's health is from subsequent infection of the puncture wounds arising from bites.

Behavioural treatment is unlikely to be effective in reducing this type of aggression. Overall, synthetic progestagens have been found to reduce fighting in 75% of cases (Hart & Hart, 1985). Though it is likely that they are particularly effective in reducing inter-male aggression, they will only be effective for the period of prescription. As soon as such drugs are withdrawn, the cat's original competitiveness towards other toms will return. Given the potentially serious side effects of these drugs, a **fighting cat's interests might be better served by agreeing with the owners of local rival cats a time-budgeting system of access to shared outdoor territories** and by prompt treatment of infected wounds.

## SOCIAL AGGRESSION BETWEEN CATS SHARING A HOUSE

Sometimes, in multi-cat households, one cat may take a dislike to one or more of the others. It will growl or hiss at its victims on sight. It may even mount, attack or pursue them aggressively out of the room or the house at nearly every encounter. Such aggression is commonly referred to as "territorial" aggression, but this term makes a questionable assumption about the aggressor's motivation. The aggressor may attack only one cat in a multi-cat household and, while the victim is usually a newcomer, it may, on occasion, be a cat with which the aggressor has previously lived on good terms. Such disputes most commonly arise when either cat reaches maturity, at about 8 – 18 months of age. The victim may become withdrawn and fearful, taking refuge outdoors or in inaccessible corners of the house. Alternatively, it may develop a strategy of defensive aggression to deal with the threat and serious fights may occur, resulting in injury.

It is important to distinguish this type of aggression from either defensive aggression (see page 48) or redirected aggression (see page 49). Aggression which builds up between two cats slowly over time, rather than erupting suddenly, is not redirected aggression. The same usually applies to attacks which, though they have a sudden onset, are directed towards a new arrival in the household. Attacks which involve chasing the victim even when it is in retreat are not defensive aggression.

This type of aggression, which is apparently prompted by intolerance of an individual cat, often does not respond adequately to treatment, possibly because it is not yet well enough understood. **Often the best and safest solution is to re-home one of the cats.** However, arranging that the cats have access, or increased access, to outdoors can be helpful in easing the tension between them. If the aggression is as serious outside as it is indoors, the cats' access times may need to be staggered. **Providing the victim with a safe haven in the house is vital** to protect it from injury and to maintain a good relationship with the owner and with any other friendly house cats. **The aggressor can then sometimes be systematically desensitized to his victim** (see page 27). The two cats should be kept apart except for supervised treatment sessions where they are exposed to each other in conditions which do not provoke hostility. Thus, to begin with, the rooms in which they are kept might be interchanged, so that the aggressor is desensitized to the smell of his victim. They then might be allowed to see each other while separated by a glass or mesh door or window. Alternatively, the cats may be placed in separate wire mesh cages where they can see each other. The cages may then be gradually brought nearer to each other as mutual tolerance increases. Feeding both cats during this exposure may improve their tolerance: the effect may be enhanced by withholding or delaying a meal to ensure that both cats are hungry before controlled introduction sessions.

**Drug treatment in the form of megestrol acetate or diazepam may be helpful**: both cats should be treated to reduce levels of arousal and so prevent the victim from developing secondary defensive aggression.

### Case history 2

*Mrs. T. sought advice about her cat Tommy, a four year old short haired male neuter. Tommy was repeatedly attacking Mrs. T.'s other cat Timothy, another short haired male neuter aged one year.*

Tommy had been acquired two years previously from a cat rescue shelter. There were no problems at this time, though Tommy was territorial towards other cats: he was allowed out of doors on demand. Mrs. T. then changed her job and had to be away from home for ten rather than seven hours per day and could not return at lunch time. To provide company for Tommy, she acquired Timothy from the same shelter. She was assured he would be friendly with other cats as he had previously lived with five other cats in a household with an elderly lady: her death had led to the cats being placed in the shelter.

From the outset, Tommy attacked Timothy ferociously on sight, biting him and mounting him aggressively. Although Timothy did not retaliate, the attacks did not abate. He received veterinary treatment several times for bite and scratch wounds. Mrs. T. tried giving both cats more attention. As this had no effect, she was forced to keep them in separate rooms and let them out alternately.

To treat the problem, Mrs. T. was advised to put Timothy in a wire cage and allow Tommy into the same room for frequent short periods, supervised by Mrs. T. Although Timothy did not react to Tommy's presence, on the first few occasions Tommy tried to attack as usual. Thwarted by the mesh of the pen, he then sat nearby, staring menacingly at Timothy and growling. If Timothy moved, Tommy hissed and advanced threateningly. If Tommy seemed particularly aggressive in any session, that session was terminated. The cats' food was divided into six meals; they were fed only in each other's presence, Timothy in the pen and Tommy outside, with his food dish moved progressively closer to the pen. Tommy was also given 2.5 mg Ovarid on alternate days for one week. The dose was then halved for a second week and halved again for a third.

The introduction procedure with Timothy in the pen was repeated in different rooms in the house. Timothy was allowed to wander freely around the house when Tommy was out. The intensity of Tommy's reactions towards Timothy declined and Timothy was allowed out of the pen with Tommy in the room at feeding times. If Timothy moved suddenly, Tommy would still hiss and stare at him. However he did not attack but would continue eating. At such times, Mrs. T. petted only Tommy, paying attention to Timothy when Tommy was elsewhere.

After three weeks, the two cats were able to share all rooms in the house without Tommy becoming aggressive. After two months, the cats would eat next to each other from separate bowls and lie close to each other by the living room fire. If one accidentally touched the other while stretching, however, Tommy would hiss at Timothy. They both used their outdoor territory simultaneously though they were never seen in each other's company outside.

## DEFENSIVE AGGRESSION

Defensive aggression occurs when the cat perceives itself to be under a threat from which it cannot escape. This threat may come from dogs, people or from other cats. This type of aggression may be recognised by the typical body postures which accompany it (see page 23). Also, the defensively aggressive cat only attacks when approached: it does not seek out the source of the threat nor pursue it if it withdraws.

Sometimes the nature of the perceived threat is obvious, as when the cat is attacked by a dog or another cat. Sometimes the object of the attack is harmless (e.g. a startling noise) and the aggression is a phobic reaction (see page 26). As mentioned above, defensive aggression can complicate other problems of aggression. Complex problems can also arise with, for example, two cats becoming defensively aggressive towards each other. This may begin when one cat inadvertently startles another or when both are exposed to the same external threat which both perceive as originating from the other. **Defensive aggression should be treated in the same way as phobias** (see page 53), with systematic desensitization and supportive drug therapy if required.

**Defensive aggression is probably the commonest type of aggression observed in the veterinary consulting room**, and most likely to be encountered when the practitioner tries to approach or restrain the cat or to carry out some uncomfortable procedure. While most investigations are relatively quick and carry little risk of long term behavioural impact on the cat, the risk to the veterinary surgeon and nursing staff can be high. Any attempt to "dominate" the defensively aggressive cat is entirely inappropriate (see page 25) and will only exacerbate the problem on the cat's next visit to the surgery. Instead, **the cat should be approached in as non-threatening and slow a manner as possible** and restrained gently but firmly. Specialised muzzles which hood the cat can have a calming effect. These should be fitted by the owner in the waiting room or even at home before setting off for the surgery. In addition, placing the cat on a piece of carpet on the examination table and pulling it slightly backwards will encourage it to take hold of it with its claws and keep them safely occupied during dorsal or facial examinations. Two people are usually required for speed of treatment, however.

## REDIRECTED AGGRESSION

Many instances in which a cat is reported to attack a person or other cat for no reason turn out to be cases of redirected aggression i.e. the cat, aroused to aggression by one stimulus, attacks another irrelevant person or cat. It does so because the original stimulus is no longer present or because it cannot be attacked. In a study by Chapman & Voith (1990) of 14 cases of aggression redirected onto people, the commonest arousing stimulus was the sight of another cat. The owner might be attacked when he approached his cat while it watched another cat through a window or if he tried to intervene in a fight between two cats. In four cases the arousing stimulus was a high-pitched noise and, in four other cases, attacks were due to the arrival of a visitor to the house. The state of arousal which gives rise to a cat's redirected aggression may persist for some time after the disappearance of the arousing stimulus (for 30 minutes or more in 6 of the 14 cases).

Several factors may further complicate the clinical picture. Redirected aggression may become classically conditioned to the victim. It may then be elicited repeatedly by the presence of the victim and in the absence of any arousing stimulus. If a cat is the victim, it may, in turn, develop a fear of the attacking cat and become defensively aggressive towards it. If the victim is the owner or other person, he or she may retaliate so strongly that the attacking cat develops a fear of him and becomes defensively aggressive towards him.

To treat this type of aggression, **the arousing stimulus must be identified so that**, in some cases, it can be eliminated. For example, if the cat becomes aroused by the sight of other cats looking in at the window, it may be possible to prevent them from passing close to the window by blocking access; it may be possible to deter them from jumping on the window sill by putting unstable objects on it. Alternatively the resident cat might be prevented from seeing outdoors by screening part of the window. If the arousing stimulus cannot be removed, the cat should be systematically desensitized to it: for example, the cat might be habituated to the arrival and presence of visitors using an indoor pen. Secondary problems in the form of phobias or defensive aggression should also be treated.

Even when the problem is successfully treated, the owner should be on the alert for a similar reaction to another arousing stimulus in the future. In this event, she should keep people and other cats away from the aggressive cat until it has calmed down. This may take some hours.

## Case history 3

*Mr and Mrs B. sought help because their three-year-old domestic short-haired cat, Bobby, was attacking Mr B. It attacked Mr B. whenever he approached it, but these attacks were most ferocious and unnerving at night: Bobby slept on the B.'s bed and attacked Mr B. whenever he approached the bed or tried to get into it.*

*Bobby and his brother Benjie lived indoors most of the time, only going into the garden with their owners for supervised excursions. About six months previously, however, Bobby had wandered off on his own, probably into the garden of a neighbour who had recently acquired a dog. He returned from this excursion suddenly and quickly, in a state of agitation, and, on entering the house, immediately attacked Benjie. He attacked his brother repeatedly over the next few days, but Mrs B. managed to treat the problem successfully on her own with what amounted to a systematic desensitization programme. She kept the cats apart most of the time, but fed them on either side of a glass door, which she gradually opened as Bobby's hostility died down.*

*The problem recurred six weeks later when Mr B.'s sister came to stay, although on this occasion they could not pin-point any specific precipitating incident. When Mr B. tried to rescue Benjie from one of Bobby's attacks, Bobby turned on him instead. Since then, Bobby's tendency to attack Mr B. had decreased somewhat; Benjie tolerated and even showed affection towards Mr B., as long as Mr B. stayed in one place. If Mr B. approached him, he would growl, spit and eventually spring at him. When he did this, Mr B. sometimes shouted at him, but never retaliated physically. In the consulting room, Mr B. was restless, pursuing Bobby behind filing cabinets, making clucking noises as he did towards Bobby at home "to try and make friends with him".*

*The most likely explanation of Bobby's behaviour was redirected aggression, initially onto Benjie and then on to Mr B. On the first occasion, the aggression was probably caused by an encounter with the neighbouring dog. The cause of the aggression in the second episode was more obscure, but probably connected with Mr B.'s sister.*

*The systematic desensitization of Bobby to Benjie seemed to be progressing satisfactorily and the B.'s were advised to continue with this approach. They were helped to devise a similar programme to desensitize Bobby to Mr B. To begin with, Mr B. was to avoid approaching Bobby but allow Bobby to come to him. Other family members were to ignore Bobby, to increase Mr B.'s attractiveness as a source of affection for him. As Bobby's confidence increased, Mr B. was to start approaching him again, gradually decreasing the distance between them, providing Bobby showed no signs of hostility.*

*It seemed likely that Bobby might show similar episodes of redirected aggression in the future. All family members, including Benjie, were to be kept away from him if he seemed roused. They were also to keep a supply of diazepam in the house and, if another episode another episode occurred, immediately to give Bobby a high enough dose to suppress the aggression (even to the point of sedation). The dosage would then be gradually reduced.*

## AGGRESSION DURING PETTING

Some cats, while being petted or stroked, will suddenly attack their owners, usually biting a hand or a wrist. Because the attack is not anticipated, often at a time when the owner is relaxing with the cat, he may feel shocked and upset out of proportion to the degree of injury inflicted.

For most cats, there is a limit to the amount of physical contact that they will tolerate in the form of being hugged, picked up or petted. When the limits of this tolerance are reached, the cat usually reacts by attempting to escape, but occasionally reacts with aggression. **Certain types of handling elicit such defensive aggression** more quickly than others, for example tickling the abdomen or chest, especially if the cat is upside down. Such handling is best avoided in favour of stroking the head and back of an upright cat.

**Owners should also be encouraged to find other ways of interacting with their cats,** for example, by playing with them. Most show some warning signs of impending attack, typically by restlessness or tail twitching. An owner who has been surprised by these attacks may be able to avoid them by detecting these signs if he is alerted to them. Ideally, however, he should always stop petting the cat before this point is reached so that it may then be possible to systematically desensitize it to the aspects of petting which it finds threatening and gradually raise its threshold of tolerance. For cats with particularly low thresholds of aggression when petted, it is advisable to cease all attempts to pick them up. Instead they should be to accustomed to being touched while feeding, standing on a firm surface such as a table. The cat can then be stroked along the back and up the tail, if this is raised in greeting. It can then be gently and slowly lifted to the floor once it has finished eating. Eventually it should come to tolerate being lifted and held off the ground, and then being cradled in an upright position while the stroking continues.

## Case History 4

*George was a nine month old male neuter Burmese kitten owned by Mr. and Mrs. G. He was an affectionate cat which frequently demanded attention from the G.'s and their friends. However he was liable to change suddenly from being relaxed and enjoying a cuddle to becoming highly active and aggressive.*

*The family had already learned to limit their petting of George to frequent short encounters and immediately to put him down as soon as he stopped purring. Otherwise he was liable to swipe at their faces with his forepaws, with claws extended. When they put him on the floor, however, George was liable to turn and attack their legs instead. The frequency of this behaviour was increasing: he had also started to stalk them at other times and to demand activity and play from them.*

*The family were advised to keep their physical contact with George to frequent short encounters, never attempting to pick him up unless they were sure he was relaxed. They were to respond to friendly demands for contact, but with stroking and caressing only. If George became aggressive or forceful in his demands for attention, the family were to hiss at him and walk away into another room. If he attacked their legs and a hiss failed to deter or distract him, they were to direct a jet of water at him. Alternatively they might distract him by dropping a bunch of keys near him. They were then to roll a ball of crumpled newspaper or one of his mouse toys past him. Thus his aggression or excitement was always met with a withdrawal of contact and his excitement was directed onto an inanimate object. Once George was calm, affectionate contact could then be renewed.*

*George's tendency to become aggressively over-excited decreased markedly under this regime. It improved further as he matured and spent more time outdoors hunting. After returning from excursions lasting many hours, he was able to relax and enjoy longer periods of affectionate contact with the family. He would occasionally lash out but the family dealt with this by dropping him to the floor and ignoring him for a few minutes.*

## IDIOPATHIC (MOTIVELESS) AGGRESSION

Occasionally a cat will mount a severe attack on its owners for no identifiable reason. In the United Kingdom this kind of behaviour is most frequently reported in Burmese cats living permanently indoors. However, the veterinary surgeon should be reluctant to accept at face value an owner's account of motiveless aggression. Before diagnosing it as such, he should look for an environmental cause or trigger. **Many cases of seemingly unpredictable aggression are, in reality, cases of defensive or redirected aggression**. He should also, of course, investigate possible physical pathology. However, where aggression is a symptom of physical disorders (e.g. neurological or endocrinological conditions, idiosyncratic dietary intolerance), additional signs will usually be evident.

If, even after investigation, the aggression remains unexplained and unpredictable, euthanasia may be the only solution. However, the fact that many cases of such aggression involve cats which live exclusively indoors suggests that **under-stimulation may be a contributory factor**.

The lack of opportunity to engage in much play or any real predatory behaviour may so increase the motivation for this type of activity that a minimal stimulus will trigger it. In such cases, it is worth trying to reduce the aggression by allowing the cat out of doors, or, where this is impossible, enriching the indoor environment through frequent provision of novel objects and increased opportunity for play.

## FURTHER READING

BORCHELT P. L. and VOITH V. L. (1987). Aggressive behaviour in cats. *Compendium Continuing Education Practicing Veterinarian*, 9, 49-56.

CHAPMAN B. L. (1991) Feline aggression: classification, diagnosis and treatment. *Veterinary Clinics of North America*, 21, 315-328.

# NEUROTIC DISORDERS

Chapter Nine _____

## MONOSYMPTOMATIC PHOBIAS

A maladaptive fear or phobia does not usually pose a real problem for cat or its owner. For example, if a cat runs out of the room when someone sneezes and returns half an hour later, neither the quality of its life nor the lives of its owners are greatly impaired. Occasionally a phobia can have a more serious impact, however: for example when a cat becomes afraid to go outside or is consistently fearful of a family member.

If possible, **the cause of the phobia should be identified**, as it may still be present. The cat may be afraid to go out because of the presence of a new cat or dog in the neighbourhood or because of building works next door. A feared family member may be startling the cat inadvertently or perhaps even punishing it for some unwanted behaviour. It should always be borne in mind that a fear response, classically conditioned to the original traumatic stimulus, may generalise in time to other similar stimuli. Thus a cat originally frightened by one person's punishing actions may steadily become fearful of more and more people.

**The first step in treatment is to eliminate the original cause of the phobia**. Alternatively, treatment may have to wait until the cause removes itself, for example, when building works on a neighbouring house are completed or until a feared relative's visit comes to an end. **The treatment of choice is systematic desensitization** (see page 27). Before starting, as much information as possible should be gathered about the attributes of the stimulus which cause the fear. For example, in the case of a cat with agoraphobia, some parts of the garden may be more frightening than others; some times of day may be more alarming, such as when children pass on the street on their way home from school. For a cat which is afraid of a person, proximity is likely to increase fear, and other factors, such as whether the person is moving as opposed to sitting still, may also be relevant. Such information will make it possible to construct a stimulus hierarchy. The cat is then exposed to the mildest stimulus in the hierarchy while in as calm a state as possible. In some instances, feeding or petting the cat will reduce anxiety sufficiently; in others it may be necessary to use medication to assist relaxation. A pen or cage can be useful as it forces the cat to confront the mild version of the phobic stimulus presented to it long enough for habituation to take place. In addition, the protection afforded by the bars of the pen may lower the cat's anxiety by providing it with a feeling of security.

If the feared object is a family member, other family members should pay the cat as little attention as possible, leaving the feared person as the sole source of food and social interaction. If visitors are feared, it may be helpful if they also offer food, but they should not do this too actively nor too early in the treatment regime.

## GENERALISED NERVOUSNESS

**For some cats, nervous, fearful behaviour may become a way of life.** They may habitually adopt a frightened body posture (crouching, tail held low, slow movements) and spend much of the day hiding behind or under furniture. When out in the open, the cat is often highly reactive and easily prompted to flight. Events which would be interesting to other cats, such as rustling leaves or a larder door being opened, may trigger a dash for cover.

**Genetic factors probably play a part in many such cases. Frequently, however, deficits in the early environment are also apparent.** As a kitten, the fearful cat may have been exposed to a restricted range of sights and sounds and thus be psychologically illequipped to cope with novelty. Sometimes, a litter may develop normally except for one kitten, which becomes progressively less confident than the rest. Its littermates are always quicker to investigate a new object or person thus denying it the opportunity to habituate to new experiences.

**Generalised nervousness of this kind usually does not improve spontaneously**. Untreated, such cats tend to become more reactive and fearful with time. Owners should therefore be encouraged to take positive steps to treat this problem as early as possible. It is usually impractical to desensitize the cat to each feared stimulus individually, as there are so many of them. The best method is often to install the cat in a cage for much of the day where it feels secure. As it becomes habituated to its surroundings, the cage can be gradually moved to less and less secluded locations. If necessary, the cat's anxiety can be reduced by covering most of the cage with a sheet or rug to provide extra initial security: this can then be removed in stages. Diazepam may also be useful, with the dose being gradually reduced before the cat becomes habituated to the drug. The combination of phenobarbitone and propranolol outlined on page 43 has also been used with some success.

## OVEREXCITEMENT, DISPLACEMENT ACTIVITIES AND STEREOTYPIES

Cats may react to stress, conflict and frustration with various forms of hyperactivity such as frequent vocalisation, restlessness or climbing curtains. Such behaviours are usually more annoying than alarming to the owners. Occasionally, however, a cat may give both owner and veterinary surgeon more cause for concern if the behaviour seems bizarre, causes harm to the cat or appears to be a symptom of organic pathology.

**The commonest of these reactions is over grooming**. Many cats lick their flanks or back as a displacement activity when faced with a mildly upsetting or confusing situation. In some cats this develops into a stereotypy, the action being repeated so often that hair may be lost and the skin surface traumatised: lick granulomas may develop. Such over grooming may also aggravate or prolong a dermatitis with medical causes. Less commonly, polydipsia and polyphagia may become stereotypic activities and, if they are initially symptoms of physical disease, they may continue as stereotypies even after successful medical treatment.

**Locomotor stereotypies** include flicking the head, freezing and chasing non-existent objects or the cat's own tail. Some of these activities are often so bizarre or the cat seems so out of touch with its surroundings that a diagnosis of epilepsy is made. Organic pathology of this kind is unlikely, however, if the cat is neither ataxic nor uncoordinated in its movements nor if it can be distracted or physically prevented from engaging in the behaviour.

Although, as mentioned in chapter 4, the causes and mechanisms of stereotypies are not fully understood, there is probably a genetic predisposition in many cases. **In addition, the stereotypy is usually triggered by some form of conflict or stress.** When excited or frustrated, many cats perform meaningless actions for a short time, such as pouncing or tail chasing. Various factors probably cause these activities to be extended and ritualised so that they become stereotypies e.g. the stress may be severe or prolonged; the activity may be reinforced by the owner's attention or the owner's reaction to the behaviour, alternating as it often does between over-solicitude and exasperation, may in itself become a further source of causative stress. In addition, as discussed in chapter 4, many stereotypies seem to be self rewarding to the cat.

The first step in the treatment of stereotypies and other forms of over-excitement is to identify and, if possible, **eliminate any sources of environmental stress.** The owner should also provide the cat with as much opportunity as possible to engage in other activities. For example, a cat which enjoys going outdoors should be allowed out as much as possible. The owner should behave consistently towards the cat and organise an ordered regime which includes a great deal of social interaction. He should not punish or startle the cat. **The abnormal behaviour should be ignored.**

Under this regime, the frequency of some over-excited behaviours will decline. **However, because of the self rewarding nature of many stereotypies, some may well persist even when sources of stress have been removed, albeit at a reduced intensity or frequency.** In these cases, the owners should be encouraged to observe closely the circumstances in which the behaviour occurs and how it begins. They may then be able to predict, at least to some extent, when it will occur: for example, before a meal, or at certain times in the evening. If so, **they should distract the cat at times of risk** by encouraging it to engage in other rewarding activities, such as play or feeding. **Even if they cannot predict the stereotypy at all, being alert to how it normally begins means that they can often successfully distract the cat at this point** by calling its name or making a mildly startling noise and then diverting its attention onto another rewarding activity.

In severe cases, medication may be necessary. In most cases, the drug of first choice is diazepam at a dosage of 1-5mg/cat b.i.d. It has been noted (McKeown, personal communication) that 20% of cats show an initial paradoxical response of excitement to this drug. This is not dose related, however, and disappears within about five days. Other drugs which have been successful in controlling stereotypies are amitriptyline (0.5-1 mg/kg b.i.d) and the long-acting morphine antagonist naltrexone. The response to anticonvulsants is usually disappointing.

## Case History 5

*Mr. & Mrs. P. sought help with the behaviour of Poirot, their four-year-old domestic short-haired male neuter, who was constantly attacking his own tail. Mr. & Mrs. P. were a childless couple in their thirties and, for most of Poirot's life, Mrs. P. had worked at home. Shortly before the behaviour began, she had started to work away from home. She was finding this difficult and stressful because of the travelling involved. At around the same time, their neighbours had acquired a new dog.*

*The behaviour had begun about four weeks previously and its frequency was increasing. Mr. P. made a video film in which Poirot could be seen moving normally around the house. From time to time, he froze, moved his head sideways and began to growl. After a few seconds, he would pounce on his own tail, then relapse into growling. These bouts of growling and pouncing lasted about five seconds and were interspersed with periods of normal movement.*

*A week before the consultation, the referring veterinary surgeon had prescribed diazepam. This had reduced the frequency of the behaviour, but made Poirot sleepy. Normally, Poirot had enjoyed* free access to the outdoors via a cat flap but, recently, the P.s had only allowed him out under supervision. This restriction seemed to be partly based on a fear that he might fall off a wall or out of a tree because of the behaviour itself or because of the influence of the diazepam, but also on a feeling that Poirot was now an invalid who could not be trusted to look after himself.

There were strong indications that Poirot's behaviour was stress related. Although it was possible that it had started as a form of redirected aggression, perhaps following an attack by the neighbour's dog, by the time the P.'s sought help it had acquired stereotypic features in that it had become repetitive and ritualised.

Mr. & Mrs. P. were clearly very attached to Poirot and extremely worried by his behaviour. They were therefore reassured that it was unlikely to be a symptom of organic disease and that it could probably be more appropriately viewed as a bad habit to which Poirot had become addicted. They were urged to protect Poirot from their own anxiety and not to treat him as an invalid. They were to allow him free access to the outdoors and were encouraged to play with him more, experimenting to find games which he particularly enjoyed. They were never to reward stereotypic behaviour but to reward normal behaviour through frequent petting.

The P.'s reported that the stereotypy occurred at greatest intensity in the morning and evening, before feeding and after supper, when the P.'s were relaxing in front of the television. Armed with this information, the P.'s were to try, if possible, to prevent the behaviour by engaging Poirot in play at these times of risk. In addition, it seemed from the video recording that the behaviour was typically preceded by freezing. They were to distract him when he froze and again engage him in play. The dosage of diazepam was to be reduced to the point at which Poirot was not unduly sleepy, but which still controlled the stereotypy.

The P.'s were told that they could not expect the stereotypy to disappear immediately but, if the treatment regime was correct, its frequency should quickly begin to decline and that this decline should be maintained. They were also advised that, if the frequency increased again in the future, perhaps as the result of some stressful experience, the problem should be treated in the same way.

Three weeks later, the referring veterinary surgeon reported that the behaviour had indeed improved and that the P.'s were much relieved. Four months later, the P.'s wrote to say that it had ceased entirely when they moved house.

The more firmly a stereotypy is established, the more difficult it is to treat. Therefore, if a behaviour has stereotypic features, it is important to institute treatment at once, even if the problem also requires medical investigation or treatment at the same time: the two approaches are not incompatible. Many cases of dermatitis involving self-mutilation fall into this category.

## FURTHER READING

CHAPMAN B. L. (1991) Feline aggression: classification, diagnosis and treatment. *Veterinary Clinics of North America*, **21**, 315-328.

VOITH V. L. and BORCHELT P. L. (1985). Fears and phobias in companion animals. *Compendium on Continuing Education for the Practicing Veterinarian*, **7**,209-217

LUESCHER U. A., MCKEOWN D. B. and HALIP J. (1991). Stereotypic or obsessive- compulsive disorders in dogs and cats. *Veterinary Clinics of North America* **21**, 401-415.

# INAPPROPRIATE URINATION AND DEFAECATION

Chapter Ten

Inappropriate urination and defaecation is the commonest kind of behaviour problem presenting in cats. Before devising a plan of treatment for an individual case, it is essential to determine the type of urination or defaecation involved.

## FAILURE OF HOUSE TRAINING

In this type of behaviour, the cat urinates or defaecates normally, but in a place unacceptable to the owner, either indoors for a cat expected to eliminate outside or, in the case of an indoor cat, away from the litter tray. Urine or faeces is deposited in normal amounts, usually on the floor, though there is often a location or substrate preference: doormats are often favoured, as are carpets in the corners of rooms or under tables.

This behaviour seems to occur with equal frequency in males and females (Olm & Houpt, 1988; Neville, 1990). In the United Kingdom, however, it seems to be more common in long haired breeds (Neville, 1991).

For most cats, house training begins at around 4 weeks of age, when kittens begin to dig and eliminate in litter provided by the breeder. Most cats instinctively play, scrape and dig in any loose rakeable material, without observing or being taught by their mother. The behaviour soon becomes more firmly established as a learned connection is formed between elimination behaviour on the one hand and the location and substrate on the other.

A few cats (among which long haired strains seem to be over-represented) do not spontaneously exhibit the digging behaviour which initiates this learning sequence. Some may respond to gentle encouragement from the owner in manipulating the kitten's paws in the litter after a meal. For others it may be necessary to confine them in a pen in which the whole floor area, other than the bed, is covered with litter. The kitten is then forced to eliminate in the litter and a learned association should then be formed. The area covered with litter is then gradually reduced. The space now left uncovered may initially be filled with tubs of dry food to discourage further elimination there. Eventually a tray with low sides is used to contain the litter; a more suitable container can be substituted later.

Some domesticated feral cats are difficult to house train because they have been accustomed since kittenhood to eliminating on concrete or hard packed soil. Some may respond to the method just described. However, **most cats presenting with a house training problem have been successfully house trained at some time in the past. In these cases, it is necessary to determine and tackle the cause of the breakdown.** A cat with a gastrointestinal or urinary tract infection may be forced to eliminate before it can reach a litter tray or garden and this behaviour may persist as a learned habit even after these functions have returned to normal. Where there is a possibility that increased frequency of urination or defaecation may lead to loss of house training, it may be advisable to confine the cat to a more restricted area (e.g. a small room such as the bathroom) containing a litter tray. This will ensure that the cat has ready access to a litter tray and will prevent the learning of an undesirable association. Other physical disabilities may make the trip outside or to a litter tray too uncomfortable or tiring for the cat; the solution is simply to provide more litter trays.

For outdoor cats, fear of leaving the house may result in a failure of house training. A new cat or dog being brought into the neighbourhood is a common cause of such fear, but single traumatic incidents, such as a near miss with a car, may occasionally lead to such problems. Similarly, indoor cats may be deterred from using the litter tray and experimentation may be necessary to determine which aspect of its environment is aversive. The following possibilities should be considered:

### Location of tray
Cats are often reluctant to eliminate in a tray which is too close to their food dish. They may also be unhappy to use a tray in a busy or public area of the house. If the tray cannot be moved, a covered tray may be more acceptable. Conversely, the cat may form a location preference for the habitual site of a litter tray, a preference which may persist when the tray is moved. The easiest solution is to replace the tray in its original position.

### Litter aversion
**Cats tend instinctively to prefer certain kinds of litter. Perhaps because of the cat's semi-desert ancestry, litters with fine grained, sand-like particles tend to be preferred** (Borchelt, 1991; Neville, 1990). Cats also learn by classical conditioning to associate the act of elimination with the feel underfoot of a certain substrate. The learned association to the litter tray may therefore be broken if a new brand of litter is introduced, especially if it is also instinctively disliked. Some may dislike brands made of compressed wood pellets, those which contain chlorophyll or which release deodorising scents when damp. Some of these deodorising agents can also cause inflammation and cornification of the soft pawpads of cats kept permanently indoors: this may lead to an aversion to using the litter. Litter trays may also become aversive if they are not cleaned often enough, though cats vary enormously in their tolerance of tray hygiene. Some will use a tray once only, while others will happily use it when almost saturated with urine. Smells often build up more quickly to an unacceptable level in a covered tray.

A cat with a mild aversion to the litter may still use its tray, but may stand on the edge or fail to dig in the litter. It may abandon the tray altogether as the aversion increases or if a more acceptable substrate presents itself. Cats which urinate on a new bath mat or carpet may not be responding to the newness of the article, as owners often suppose, but to its superior acceptability as a substrate.

### Learned aversions
A cat may stop using its litter tray after having had an unpleasant experience there, such as being startled by a loud noise while in the act of elimination. Sometimes another family member or the family dog may take advantage of the cat's temporary immobility to trap it on the tray; an owner may pick it up from the tray in order to administer a medicine. An aversion may be further compounded if the cat is bodily placed or chased onto a litter tray which it has ceased to use. Removal of the cause of the aversion is a necessary condition of successful treatment. It is often not a sufficient condition, however, as the cat may have learned new preferences in the meantime.

For this reason, it is important to treat this kind of problem as quickly as possible, as it will become more recalcitrant with time.

**In order to reverse an undesirable learned preference, the litter tray should be made as attractive as possible by incorporating some of the features of the learned preference.** Thus, if the cat has formed the habit of urinating in a certain corner of the room, the tray should be placed there. If it has learned to prefer carpet as a substrate, a piece of carpet should initially be placed in the tray. It should then be covered with an ever increasing layer of fine litter until it is thick enough for the underlying carpet to be removed. The tray should also be made more attractive by making it smell like a tray in regular use, perhaps by adding to it a little of the inappropriate substrate containing the cat's own urine.

**At the same time, the cat should, if possible, be denied access to the other places where it has learned to eliminate.** Failing that, these places should be made less attractive. Dishes of food may be put there as few cats will eliminate where they eat. A carpet might be temporarily covered with plastic to prevent access to it and to make the surface less comfortable for the cat to walk on.

**Inappropriate elimination areas should also be thoroughly cleaned**, but not with a scented cleaner or one which is ammonia based. Such scents may attract the cat back to the same place, either instinctively or as a result of conditioning. After excess liquid has been mopped up, an enzymatic or biological cleaner should be used to remove remaining protein compounds. Surgical spirit or other alcohol may be used to dissolve fatty residues.

**The cat should not be punished for eliminating in the wrong place, even if caught in the act.** This may further stress and confuse it and cause it to eliminate in a wider variety of places.

Once the habit of eliminating in the litter tray only has been re-established, the tray can be moved to a more appropriate location by degrees and more convenient litter introduced in increasing proportions. For example, a commercial litter may gradually replace sand, which is heavy and therefore difficult to carry. At the same time, the cat may be allowed access, again on a gradual basis, to the places where inappropriate elimination previously occurred. It can be helped to view them as non-elimination areas by being fed meals or treats there.

**In some cases, a more extreme form of re-training may be necessary.** This involves confining the cat in a pen, as described on page 57 in connection with the house training of feral cats. Such treatment is unlikely to be successful unless the cause of the problem is also addressed. If being enclosed makes the cat persistently distressed, the technique is clearly inappropriate.

## Case History 6

*Mrs. MacJ., a cheerful Glaswegian, sought advice about Jock, her 5 year old domestic short haired cat, a male neuter, who often urinated and defaecated outside the litter tray.*

*Jock and Mrs. MacJ. lived in a tenement flat with two other male neutered cats. Jock had been acquired in a roundabout way: Mrs. MacJ. had taken an ill cat belonging to a neighbour to the People's Dispensary for Sick Animals  The cat had died and the PDSA had offered Jock, a 12 week old kitten to Mrs. MacJ., who had been rescued some weeks previously. The neighbour had accepted this replacement, but then rejected him when she discovered that he was not house trained. This behaviour had persisted (and been tolerated by Mrs. MacJ.) for five years. The referring veterinary surgeon had pronounced the problem to be incurable, but Mrs. MacJ. was prepared to put up with it indefinitely if necessary.*

*The other cats in Mrs. MacJ.'s flat always used the litter trays. One tray was kept permanently* in the bathroom; the other was kept in the hall but removed when visitors were expected. Jock used the trays sometimes, making a soft chattering noise which Mrs. MacJ. interpreted as protest. Mrs. MacJ. provided a litter which was composed of large particles. When Jock did not use the tray, he invariably urinated or defaecated in a corner of the hall behind the front door. If Mrs. MacJ. put tray there, he eliminated beside it.

It seemed likely that at the age when kittens normally start to eliminate away from the living area and to practice digging in a substrate, Jock had been housed in a cage which denied him that opportunity and he had not acquired a strong preference for eliminating in loose, rakeable material. He had later learned a combined substrate/location preference for carpet behind the hall door. There was also evidence that he found the litter in the trays aversive to some extent.

Fortunately, Mrs. MacJ. had an offcut of the hall carpet. It was suggested that she put a square of this in the corner where Jock habitually eliminated. The adjacent area was to be covered with plastic sheeting to discourage elimination there. Once elimination on the square of carpet was reliably established, this was to be placed in a large, low sided tray. The next step would be to sprinkle a fine, sand-like litter on the carpet, proceeding in gradual stages until the carpet was covered. The litter could then be transferred to a smaller receptacle with higher sides.

Follow up telephone calls took place at intervals of two or three weeks. Treatment proceeded more or less to plan, except that initially Jock did not urinate on the offcut square of carpet, but used a corner of the hall well away from the plastic. It seemed that this might be because the square slipped on the plastic and did not feel secure enough. However, nailing it down did not improve matters. Mrs. MacJ. then removed the plastic sheeting and this had the desired effect of inducing Jock to eliminate on the square. A further set back occurred when Mrs. MacJ.'s daughter threw away the square of carpet because it was so soiled. Fortunately, Jock accepted a piece of underfelt as a substitute. At the last contact, Jock was still eliminating away from the litter tray occasionally, but at a much reduced frequency.

## URINE MARKING

Urine marking can usually be distinguished from normal urination by the characteristic body posture of the cat (see fig 6) and the location of the marks. The cat usually stands with tail erect and sprays 1-2 ml of urine horizontally onto a vertical surface. Occasionally urine marking may be carried out in a squatting posture, but the volume of urine is still comparatively small. The most common locations for spraying are entrances to houses or rooms and routes through the house normally used by people or other cats. Items brought into the house (e.g. plastic carrier bags of shopping, new furniture) may also be sprayed. Some cats may form idiosyncratic spraying habits, targeting, for example, the elements of electric fires, electric wall sockets, washing machines or video recorders. This may be because the heat produces a smell which attracts the cat.

Many entire tom cats spray in the house, leaving a strong, characteristic smell. Although castration eliminates this behaviour in most male cats, around 10% persist. Also, about 5% of females spray indoors (Hart & Cooper, 1984): the problem seems harder to treat than in males. Spraying is more common in multi-cat households, particularly in castrated males living with female housemates (Hart & Cooper, 1984). When the cat population in a household reaches a very high density, however, spraying often seems to be suppressed. Indoor spraying also seems more prevalent in certain breeds, for example, in Siamese and Burmese cats (Neville, 1993). This may be related to the greater emotional reactivity of these breeds (see page 71).

Urine marking is only one of various kinds of scent marking behaviour, all of which are part of the cat's normal repertoire (see Chapter 3). In fact, most outdoor cats of both sexes, neutered or entire, spray urine outside. The function of scent marking is not fully understood. A commonly held view is that it is employed as a territorial mark to deter intruders. Certainly, a cat may start

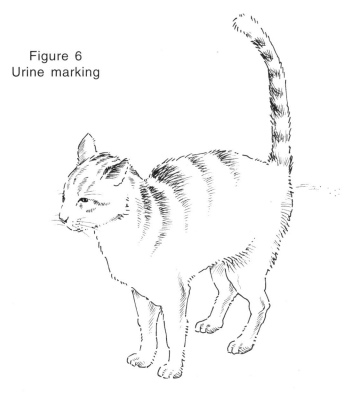

Figure 6
Urine marking

to spray more frequently outdoors and even indoors when a new cat arrives in the household or neighbourhood. The installation of a cat flap may have the same effect, presumably because indoors is then perceived as continuous with outdoors. It may also be triggered if a new person or pet of another species joins the household. However, other cats do not typically retreat from or avoid spray marks; they usually approach them and sniff. They sometimes show the Flehmen reaction: they then may or may not mark over them. Also, spraying may occur in circumstances where there is no territorial threat. Cats may spray when frustrated: if, for instance, the owner suddenly breaks off social contact or fails to respond to the cat's attention-seeking behaviour.

It may therefore be most accurate, in the present state of knowledge, to view the function of spraying as increasing a cat's own sense of security in the face of either a territorial challenge or another stressor (Neville, 1990). It has also been suggested (Cooper & Hart, 1992) that because spraying in some cats is suppressed by progestagens and in others by diazepam, two separate neural and motivational systems may influence spraying behaviour: one related to sexual behaviour and the other to anxiety. In some cases, the behaviour also seems to be maintained by instrumental learning, with attention from the owner acting as a reward.

## Treatment

Owners often instinctively try to deal with the problem of indoor urine spraying by punishing the cat. As ever, **punishment not delivered at the time is completely ineffective (see page 18); contemporaneous punishment (e.g. shouting, smacking) usually makes the spraying habit more secretive**. There is also a danger that milder interventions (e.g. remonstrating with the cat) may even act as a reward. More ingenious and sophisticated forms of remote punishment are sometimes advocated. For example, it is sometimes suggested that the owner hide and fire a water pistol at the spraying cat or that mouse traps or cap bangers are placed at favourite spraying places. It has even been suggested that electrified tin foil be placed at the site so that spraying causes an electric shock to be delivered to the cat's hind quarters. These measures are likely to increase the cat's stress level and so increase the frequency of spraying. Even if they are effective as a deterrent, they are likely to prompt the cat merely to move its spraying site. Such approaches should therefore be avoided.

Less stressful deterrents are sometimes advocated. Pepper or other substances marked for the purpose may deter some cats from spraying in specific places. Aluminium foil (not electrified) or trays of marbles or pine cones (which are uncomfortable to stand on) placed at the base of the site may have the same effect. These measures are unlikely to cause a deterioration in the situation: on the other hand, they are likely merely to displace the spraying to another location. **A manoeuvre which is more often successful is placing food at the base of the spraying site** as cats are extremely reluctant to spray their own food. Dry food is best: it lasts longer when loose and it can even be stuck to the dish to prevent it being eaten. Its superior efficacy is probably due to the fact that food is reassuring rather than alarming and gives the cat a feeling of security at places where it feels under threat. Even if no deterrents are placed at spraying posts, it is important that the marks be cleaned in the way described on page 59.

**The main aim of the therapeutic regime should be to reduce the perceived threat to the cat and make it feel more secure in its territory.** In some cases, this can be achieved by boarding up the cat flap so that the inside is no longer perceived as continuous with the outside and neighbouring cats can no longer invade the core territory. It may also be helpful to block the cat's view from the window, so that it cannot see neighbouring cats. Threats to security within the household, such as new animal or human arrivals, may be impossible to remove. In many cases, too, there may not be a single obvious threat but the cat's behaviour may be the result of the cumulative effect of several events. **Where the sources of stress cannot be removed or even fully identified, the cat should be provided with a small core territory within the house** to which it can safely retreat when threatened. Where it is suspected that the spraying is being rewarded by the owner's reaction, the behaviour should, if possible, be ignored. Owners should be prepared for an initial increase in the frequency of spraying before it starts to decline (see page 17).

Cases which do not respond to behavioural measures alone may require drug support. Diazepam is equally likely to be effective in males and females. A dose of 1-2mg/cat daily for three to four weeks, followed by a gradual reduction in dosage is recommended. If spraying resumes, a low maintenance dose may be necessary. A combination of propranolol and phenobarbitone (page 43) may be helpful in some cases. Treatment with progestagens carries a higher risk of side effects but may be effective in cats which do not respond to anxiolytics. Megestrol acetate, at a dose of 2.5mg/cat on alternate days for one week followed by two weeks on a gradually reducing dosage, is more likely to be helpful to male cats and to cats in single cat households (Hart, 1980). In some cases it may be necessary to administer a low dose for an indefinite period: in view of possible side effects (see page 42) this is a regime of last resort. Drug therapy should always be used as a support to behavioural treatment: it is unlikely to effect a cure on its own.

Surgical methods have been found to be effective in cats unresponsive to behavioural or drug treatment. (Hart, 1982) found that olfactory tractotomy eliminated spraying in 11 out of 16 cats: spayed females responded better than castrated males. Eger (1988) found it successful in three out of three cats. Transient anorexia (presumably due to anosmia) was the only significant side effect. More recently, bilateral ischiocavernosus myectomy was carried out on ten castrated, spraying males (Komtebedde & Hauptman, 1989). Four months later, spraying was eliminated in five cases and reduced in three. The authors suggest that spraying may be reduced because the cat cannot erect and extend the penis or because it cannot aim the urine at a particular area. Such interventions, however, must significantly reduce the cat's quality of life: other measures, including rehoming, are always preferable.

## Case history 7

*Nicky was a two year old male neutered Birman owned by Miss N. Over the previous six months he had been spraying in the house with increasing frequency. He sprayed all over the house* indiscriminately, especially in the sitting room and in Miss N.'s bedroom when he managed to gain access to it.

The other human occupant of Miss N.'s house was her boyfriend who stayed there intermittently. Nicky's spraying was not affected by his presence: in fact the only room where Nicky did not spray was the spare room where Miss N.'s boyfriend kept some equipment and worked when he stayed there.

About a year previously, a stray female cat, Daisy, had taken up residence. Miss N. had her spayed and had intended to find another home for her. However, she seemed so settled and the prospect of finding another home seemed so remote, that Miss N. had come to regard her as a permanent resident. She spent a great deal of time outdoors and had access only to the hall. Although she and Nicky tolerated each other without aggression, they mostly avoided each other.

Miss N. bred Birmans and had two entire breeding queens: Lily (aged four) and Polly (aged 18 months). Both had raised litters in the past six months. Miss N. was certain that Nicky's spraying had not increased when the females were in oestrus; it had increased, however, once the litters were born. The reason for this became clear when it emerged that Nicky was normally accustomed to sleeping with Miss N. and to spending much of the day in her bedroom. When there were litters of kittens, however, Miss N. kept them and the mother in her bedroom and Nicky was excluded. Miss N. also devoted most of her attention to them at the expense of Nicky.

Another stressful event had occurred six months previously: Norman, Nicky's litter-mate, was killed in a road traffic accident. Miss N. lived in the country and had judged it safe to allow Nicky and Norman out. She was extremely upset by Norman's death and blamed herself. As a result, she let Nicky out much less often than before: she had supposed that, because he was the less adventurous of the two brothers, this was not a significant deprivation for him. However, she imagined that Nicky had been deeply upset by his brother's death and that this might have prompted him to start spraying.

It was suggested to Miss N. that it was more likely that Nicky's spraying was prompted by frustration: firstly at being excluded from Miss N.'s bedroom and, secondly, at being confined to the house. Miss N. was interested in these possibilities and agreed to observe Nicky's behaviour more closely in the hope of pinpointing the situations which triggered spraying. She spontaneously suggested that she should pay more attention to Nicky and perhaps allow him outdoors more. She became tearful as she talked of her conflict between her fear that he might meet the same fate as his brother and her realisation that more freedom would improve his quality of life. It was also suggested that a low dose of diazepam be prescribed for Nicky, as it seemed important that some improvement in the situation should occur quickly.

When Miss N. telephoned ten days later, it was to report that the spraying seemed to be steadily decreasing: having observed Nicky more closely, she had realised that he mostly sprayed at times when he had previously been accustomed to going outside: she now allowed him to do this. The diazepam had been discontinued after a few days, when he became ataxic.

## MIDDENING

When middening outdoors, the cat deposits faeces at the edge of its home range or on walkways shared by many cats. Indoors, the behaviour is unusual but, when it occurs, faeces are usually deposited openly near doors or on routes used by the family. Places of significance for the cat, such as beds, chairs or the tops of fridges, may also be middened. Middening is rarer than urine marking and more difficult to treat successfully. The motivation, however, appears to be the same. **The aim of treatment should therefore be to reduce stress and to provide the cat with an area where it can feel secure.**

## NERVOUS ELIMINATION

Some cats may respond to stress or anxiety by urinating or, more rarely, by defaecating. Such behaviour may be prompted by a range of stimuli: a sudden, loud noise, punishment by the owner, disruption of household routines or a sustained challenge from another house cat. Occasionally, it may be prompted by the appearance of suitcases or other objects which signal the imminent departure of the owner. It may also be triggered by the installation of new furniture or carpets.

This type of urination is usually seen in cats which are generally nervous. It can be distinguished from other forms of urination by the events which precede it and by the places where it occurs: either it will occur at random in no specific location or the cat will urinate when hiding under or behind furniture. **It should be treated in the same way as other neurotic disorders** (see Chapter 9). In some cases, for example when it occurs in response to the laying of new carpets, systematic desensitization may be appropriate. In others, where a transient stimulus can be identified (e.g. builders working in the house), it may be wiser to shield the cat from the source of its worries until the threat has passed.

## FURTHER READING

BORCHELT P. L and VOITH V. L. (1986). Elimination behaviour problems in cats. *Compendium on Continuing Education for the Practicing Veterinarian*, **8**, 197-205.

# MISCELLANEOUS PROBLEMS

Chapter Eleven _____

## SCRATCHING FURNITURE

Scratching on vertical or near vertical surfaces is essential self-maintenance behaviour for a cat. It helps to slough off the dead outer layers of the claws and maintain sharp points. Outdoor cats use tree trunks and fence posts for this purpose. Indoor cats must be provided with suitable scratching posts if furniture is to be protected.

If a cat scratches only one or two pieces of furniture, then the primary motivation is likely to be claw maintenance: the aim of treatment should be to redirect the behaviour onto a more acceptable surface. Punishment is unlikely to be effective, though an appropriately timed hiss can sometimes temporarily deter the cat and protect furniture for the time being. In the long term, redirection of unwanted scratching behaviour is best achieved by covering the scratched surface with attractive material not found anywhere else in the house: sisal or bark, rather than carpet, are appropriate. Once scratching on this surface has been established, the material can be transferred onto a scratching post. This should be placed directly in front of the targeted piece of furniture, then gradually moved to a more convenient location.

Scratching also has a territory marking function. As with indoor urine spraying, when the cat is scratching on a number of surfaces, especially near doors or walkways, the behaviour is likely to be at least partly motivated by the desire to mark territory. Measures should be taken to increase the cat's self confidence (see page 62).

In North America, scratching is sometimes prevented or treated by surgical declawing. It is obviously an effective treatment and is reported to have fewer side effects than is commonly supposed (Landsberg, 1991). Such mutilation could only be justified, however, when behaviour modification methods had failed and euthanasia of the cat was being contemplated by the owner.

## PROBLEMS OF ATTACHMENT

Cats show considerable variation in their personalities, including the degree to which they enjoy the company of people (see page 21). This is not always appreciated by inexperienced owners and may give rise to surprise or disappointment, particularly if a cat is markedly less sociable than their previous one. In addition to normal variations in degrees of attachment, however, difficulties can arise which need to be remedied, because they impair the quality of life of cat and owner.

## OVER ATTACHMENT

Over attached cats may follow their owners constantly, perhaps crying regularly in an effort to engage them in physical contact. They may become agitated or nervous when separated from the owner. Often these cats also demonstrate pronounced infantile behaviour towards their owners, such as sucking their clothes or skin. Some have never have shown normal, independent behaviour: they may, for example, develop a very close attachment to the breeder early in life and remain in her home after weaning. Over attachment may also occur after intensive nursing during illness or in old age.

Indoor cats seem more prone to become over attached to one family member on whom they are particularly dependent for stimulation and social contact. Often the relationship is a reciprocal one, with the owner strongly attached to the cat and encouraging infantile behaviour. Even owners who find their cats' over attached behaviour a nuisance may still feel guilty about rejecting their overtures or may fear losing their cats' affection if they stop responding to their demands.

### Treatment
**Increased dependence on the owner may be regarded as normal behaviour in old age and the owner should be encouraged to find compromises which are acceptable to both parties.** A cat which calls out constantly at night for company, for example, may be content if provided with a bed in the owner's bedroom. **Younger cats showing over attachment should be encouraged to lead more independent lives** and to develop new interests, both indoors and outdoors, which do not involve the owner. For example, new toys and objects may be provided indoors and in the garden for the cat to investigate and explore. At the same time, the owner should make dependent behaviour less rewarding by responding to it only briefly, if at all. Where the cat is over dependent on one particular family member, other family members should be encouraged to interact more with the cat and take on the roles of feeding, petting and playing with it.

In many cases, the chief problem may lie not in devising an appropriate treatment regime, but in persuading the owner to carry it out. Some owners encourage dependent behaviour in their cats in an attempt to deal with their own psychological problems, projecting their own dependent needs onto the cat (see page 35). In other words, some owners need to be needed, because they themselves are lonely. They may have to be tactfully persuaded that their cat's over attachment to them is not in its best interest. Reducing the dependency may be difficult because an owner may hesitate to reject the cat's advances because they imagine that the cat will be as upset as they would be. In such circumstances, it may help to point out that adult cats normally greet each other only briefly and do not engage in prolonged sucking or cuddling sessions.

Other owners may respond in a more complex and inconsistent way to their cat's dependent behaviour (see Chapter 6). They may at times encourage their cat's attachment because they 'need to be needed'; yet at others they may reject or even punish dependent behaviour because they cannot tolerate their own dependent needs or, by extension, those of others. Their cats may then develop an anxious over attachment to their owners which can prove all the more resistant to treatment. It can be difficult to empathize with such a complex mixture of feelings and reactions, but a non judgmental approach on the part of the veterinary surgeon is most likely to be successful. Owners in such circumstances may need to be encouraged to separate their feelings about their cat's behaviour from their own actions towards it. They should be helped to understand that they should neither punish nor excessively reward their cat's dependent behaviour.

## UNDER ATTACHMENT

Many cats resist being picked up and held. Some, however, dislike being even touched; a few will not even tolerate their owners' approach, especially those which started life as feral cats and had no contact with people in the early weeks of life.

Preference for play over physical contact and petting is probably a personality trait established early in life: owners must learn to adapt to this aspect of the cat's behaviour rather than attempt to modify it. Intolerance of the owner's proximity whatever the owner is doing is more likely to be due to lack of contact with people during the sensitive period (see page 31). Such a deficiency is hard to rectify completely. The treatment outlook is better for cats which have been initially socialised to people but which have become fearful of them later in life. This can happen if, for example, the owners repeatedly carry out upsetting or traumatic medical procedures such as forcing the cat to swallow pills. Other cats may be deterred by the over enthusiastic friendliness of an inexperienced owner, often a young child. Occasionally such fear can be the result of a traumatic incident such as being kicked by someone. Some stray cats which used to be pets also fall into this category.

## Treatment

In all these cases, the veterinary surgeon should explain to the owners the basic rule of cat social behaviour: that cats spend more time interacting with people who respond to them rather than those who try to initiate contact. The owners should therefore stop actively trying to make contact with their cats through chasing them or reaching out to them. They should wait passively for the cats to approach them; they should make themselves as attractive as possible to the cat by offering food or titbits, playing with toys or by lying in the cat's favourite resting places, such as in front of the fire. When the cat does approach the owner, the owner should always respond, using slow, calm movements and a soft voice. In severe cases, anxiolytics may be helpful (see page 42).

In severe cases, the cat may be penned for a short time to accustom it to close human presence. The owner should approach the cat head first to simulate cat greeting behaviour. Hands, which the cat may perceive as threatening, should be introduced later.

## PICA

**The commonest form of pica is fabric chewing**. This was first documented in the 1950s and was thought to be limited to Siamese strains. However a recent survey of 152 fabric eating cats (Neville and Bradshaw, 1992) showed the behaviour to be more widespread. Although 55% of these cats were Siamese, 28% were Burmese and 11% were cross bred cats. Males and females were equally represented and most cats began to show the behaviour at 2-8 months of age. Ninety-three per cent started by eating wool, 64% progressed to cotton and 54% also consumed synthetic fabrics.

While some fabric eaters chew or eat material on a regular basis, others do so only sporadically. Many consume large amounts of material, from sources such as woollen jumpers, cotton towels, underwear or furniture covers, without apparent harm, although surgery is required in a few cases to clear gastric obstructions and impaction of material. The damage to property, however, can be considerable.

The reasons for this behaviour are uncertain, although its greater prevalence in some Siamese and Burmese strains points to a genetic factor. One possible interpretation of the behaviour is that it is a redirected form of early suckling behaviour, a hypothesis supported by the fact that some cats cease eating fabric as they mature. Also, it is sometimes seen in cats which are over-dependent on their owners (see above), the fabric eating being triggered by separation from the owners.

Alternatively, fabric eating may be a form of a redirected prey catching and ingestion sequence. Forty per cent of the fabric eating cats in the survey had little or no access to the outdoors and hence were denied the opportunity to hunt. Also, some cats eat fabric only or chiefly at mealtimes:

if they can, they take a woollen item to the food bowl and eat it in alternate mouthfuls with their usual diet.

Fabric eating may also be a form of stereotypic behaviour. In many cats its onset is triggered by a stressful event, for example moving from the breeders to a new home or the addition of another cat to the household.

### Treatment

Remote punishment such as a jet of water from a water pistol may temporarily deter some cats, but it merely drives many to eat fabric in secret. There is also the risk of making the problem worse by increasing the level of stress on the cat.

Occasionally, however, neutralising the rewarding effect of the chewing is successful. Baiting a piece of fabric with menthol or oil of eucalyptus and leaving it available for the cat to find and chew will deter a few fabric eaters permanently.

Simply denying the cat access to any edible fabric for a few weeks may also cure the problem by breaking the habit. More often, however, it is also necessary to provide some positive outlet for the behaviour. For example, dry cat food might be made constantly available, either in addition to or instead of the usual diet. Offering the cat gristly meat attached to large bones will increase the time spent handling and eating food: this may decrease or eliminate the desire to eat fabric. Alternatively, the fibre content of wet diets may be increased by adding bran, tissues or chopped, undyed wool.

Finally, the behaviour may simply be managed in some cats by making available a supply of unwanted disposable woollen garments, especially at mealtimes. Jumble sales are a good cheap source of such material.

### Case history 8

*Mrs. M. sought help with Ming, her Siamese neutered male aged 8. Since she had acquired him as a 13 week old kitten, he had chewed bath towels, tea towels, woollen clothes and, sometimes, any fabric he could find. She had dealt with this by shutting away valuable clothes and fabrics and by denying Ming access to bedrooms.*

*Ming lived permanently indoors and was otherwise a problem free cat. His fabric eating became a nuisance only when Mr. and Mrs. M.'s first child was born and he started to chew baby clothes, nappy liners and cot bedding. It was impossible for his owners to supervise and prevent his chewing while caring for their baby at the same time.*

*To begin with, Ming was supplied with old, unwanted pieces of fabric to eat at meal times. Although this reduced his fabric eating at other times, it did not eliminate it. Next, Ming was allowed outdoors in the hope that the increase in stimulation and the opportunity to hunt and eat rodents and birds might reduce his desire to seek out fabric. Almost immediately, Ming proved to be a successful hunter and adapted well to outdoor life. He was put outdoors when the baby required attention and he could not be adequately supervised. However, within a few days, he ceased eating any fabric at all.*

*For six months he was trouble free and his owners relaxed their vigilance. Thereafter, from time to time, he engaged in bouts of fabric eating. These were usually triggered by disruptions to his routine: for example, after returning from boarding at a cattery or when there was a large number of house guests. In most cases, his owners were able to foresee these setbacks: they confined Ming to a fabric free room such as the kitchen and put him outside for long periods.*

More rarely, cats may engage in other undesirable forms of pica, for example eating rubber or chewing electric cables. In general, these problems should be treated using an approach similar to that outlined for fabric eating. If the behaviour is putting the cat's life in danger, it may be necessary first of all to use remote punishment to deter it: a cap banger (available from most joke shops) may be placed under a cable such as an aerial or hi-fi speaker wire which does not carry electric current. Alternatively, the cables may be made less attractive by smearing them with aromatic oils. The cat should be also prevented from engaging in the pica, preferably by removing the items concerned or denying access to high risk areas.

**Most cats eat plant materials from time to time**. The function of the behaviour remains obscure, although it has been suggested that its purpose is to obtain roughage, minerals, vitamins or to act as an emetic. The behaviour can be inconvenient to the owner if house plants are consumed; dangerous to the cat if the plants are toxic or if, as occasionally happens, it develops a preference for a plant with a jagged leaf. Such plants should be removed or placed out of the cat's reach. Failing that, the cat can be deterred using the remote punishment tactics described above. In addition, the cat should be provided with an alternative source of plant food, such as the tubs of seedling sprouts available from most pet shops.

A disproportionate number of cats engaging in pica seem to be single, indoor cats and boredom may be a causative factor. In these cases it may be helpful if the owners provide more toys for the cat and spend more time handling and playing with it. They might also consider acquiring a second cat as a companion.

# PREVENTION OF PROBLEMS

Chapter Twelve

Behaviour problems are easier to prevent than to cure. Although veterinary surgeons are often consulted only after a problem has developed, they are nevertheless sometimes in a position to offer advice, either to a breeder or to an owner which will stop a potential difficulty occurring.

## THE BREEDER'S RESPONSIBILITIES

Turner *et al* (1986) have demonstrated that a kitten's friendliness is correlated with the friendliness of its father. Compared with dogs, however, the direct experimental evidence for genetic influences on cat personality is slight. On the other hand, there is sufficient indirect evidence from other species and from breed differences (see page 71) which make it extremely likely that personality traits such as nervousness are influenced by genetic factors. It is therefore incumbent upon breeders to use only cats of stable temperament for breeding.

The socialisation period for cats ends at around seven weeks of age, earlier than the comparable sensitive period for dogs which ends at 12-14 weeks. The regulations of the Governing Council of the Cat Fancy dictate that breeders keep their kittens until they are 12 weeks old, long past the end of this crucial time. Cat breeders, especially those of pedigree cats, have therefore an even greater responsibility than dog breeders to ensure that their kittens are properly socialised.

Kittens should be regularly handled from birth (see page 30). When they start to move about and play, they should be provided with as interesting and complex an environment as possible. They should not be kept penned all the time, but should spend a large part of the day exposed to normal domestic sights and sounds. They should also meet a variety of people, including children.

## THE OWNER'S RESPONSIBILITIES

### Indoor versus outdoors.
The quality of life of most cats is enhanced by excursions out of doors. Some owners cannot provide this opportunity for their cats, for example, if they live in a flat. Other owners choose to restrict their cats to an indoor life for a variety of reasons: there may be dangerous roads nearby or the owners may be especially protective. For owners who can offer their cats access to the outdoors, but are uncertain whether to do so, it is a question of weighing up potential risks and benefits. The following considerations may prove helpful:

The smallest range of a feral urban cat has been found to be around 200 square metres (Tabor, 1983) which is larger than the floor space of many flats. As female cats tend to have smaller ranges than male cats, they are probably better suited to indoor life. Even so, an owner should not contemplate keeping an indoor cat unless he can provide a minimum standard of environmental and social stimulation.

In assessing quality of environment, Mertens and Schar (1988) have suggested that **a basic minimum requirement for an indoor cat is that it should not be able to see every point of its surroundings from one position without moving or searching**. In other words, that it should probably not be kept in a flat with less than two rooms. In addition, the space available to the cat should be maximised by allowing it access to as many rooms as possible, including the bathroom. The space available to it can also be increased by installing wall shelves at different heights in the room. If it is safe to do so, the cat should also be allowed access to windowsills, from which it can observe the outside world. Time spent in a secure pen in the garden will also be appreciated. The environment should be enriched by constantly providing new objects for exploration. These need not be expensive toys: cardboard boxes, packing cases, tree branches and arches made of folded newspaper, for example, will usually engage a cat's interest.

Social stimulation is also necessary. If the owners are regularly away from home for more than an hour or two at a time, they should consider acquiring two cats rather than one. It is best to acquire two cats together as kittens: for example, siblings from the same litter, than to try to introduce a second cat into the household later (see page 73).

**Choosing a breed of cat**
Although most cats (92%) in Britain are domestic shorthairs of no specific breed, the proportion of pedigree cats is increasing (Pet Food Manufacturers Association Report, 1992). As with dogs, these have the advantage that their temperaments can be predicted with more certainty than those of non-pedigree cats. Even within a breed, however, wide variations in personality are found. A scientific study of breed differences in behaviour, based either on direct observations of the cats' behaviour or on the views of owners, has yet to be carried out. In the USA, Hart (1979) has produced personality profiles for various breeds, based on an "informal" survey of show judges. In Britain, Fogle (1991) asked 100 veterinary surgeons to rank six breeds on ten personality characteristics. The drawback of both studies is that they drew on the stereotypes of "experts" rather than directly on the experience of owners of individual cats. Cat World Magazine (1992), on the other hand, invited readers to complete a questionnaire about their cats' personalities. Although this produced data based on owner observations, the sample was self selected and therefore liable to bias. However, the credibility of the results of all these studies is increased by the fact that they are more or less consistent. Six typical breed personalities which emerged:

**Siamese** seem to be affectionate, confident and attention seeking. They are active and playful, but they are also vocal and can be destructive.
**Burmese** also seem to be affectionate, confident and demanding. They cope least well with being left alone. They are also more likely to show aggression to other cats.
**Abyssinians** seem to be active and vocal, but less dependent on human company. Some may dislike being petted and may be shy and fearful of strangers.
**Persians** seem to be calm and docile: they tolerate grooming and handling well. They scored low on activity and playfulness. They are also more prone to house soiling.
**British Shorthairs** should theoretically show the greatest variation in temperament. However, they were rated as being the most tolerant of separation from the owners and most friendly with other cats.

Turner (personal communication) has recently compared Swiss owners' ratings of Siamese, Persian and mixed breed domestic shorthairs. He also made similar comparisons using direct observations of 80 cat owning households. His results largely confirm the above impressions. The purebreds were rated as more affectionate, predictable and dependent than the mixed breed cats and they spent more time interacting with their owners. The Siamese were rated as more active and playful than the Persians and spent even more time interacting with their owners. However, Turner's study also found that the Persians had fewest house soiling problems and the Siamese the most. One possible explanation of this may be connected with the type of inappropriate elimination involved i.e. spraying versus failure of house training.

Owners therefore should be encouraged to reflect on the temperament of the cat best suited to their own domestic circumstances and personality. Although, as has already been discussed, a cat's breed is no guarantee of its temperament, it is at least a useful starting point.

### Choosing a kitten

Prospective owners should find out from the breeder as much as possible about the kitten's early environment (see pages 30-31), especially in the case of a pedigree kitten which normally cannot leave the breeder until twelve weeks of age. A non-pedigree kitten can usually go to its new home as soon as it is weaned, at around six weeks of age. Kittens which have been reared in an outhouse or cattery, without exposure to people or to common domestic sights or sounds, should be avoided.

The prospective owner should observe the mother and her litter. The mother's behaviour is relevant because of her genetic influence on the kittens' behaviour. For the same reason, it is also useful to meet the father, though this is rarely possible, especially with crossbred cats. The mother's behaviour is especially important, because the kittens learn skills and social behaviour from her.

Although the personality of the adult cat cannot be predicted with certainty from observations of the kittens' behaviour, there is enough evidence that certain characteristics persist into adulthood to make such observations worthwhile. For example, vocal kittens tend to become vocal cats and kittens which try to escape when handled tend, as adults, to spend less time interacting with their owners (Karsh and Turner, 1988). There is also evidence (Moelk, 1979, Karsh, 1984) that shy, timid kittens tend to grow into shy, timid cats. Prospective owners should therefore insist on spending some time observing and handling the litter. As with different breeds of cat, kittens of different temperaments will appeal to different owners: they should be encouraged to pick a kitten with a personality which appeals to them, with the proviso that extremely shy or timid kittens should be left to experienced owners. Others who take on these kittens with the aim of curing or rescuing them may well be doomed to disappointment.

### Introducing a kitten into the household

If there are already cats in the household, care must be taken to ensure that the kitten is accepted by them. The kitten should already be eliminating reliably in the litter tray. If not, steps should be taken without delay to house train it (see page 57). All kittens should be kept indoors for a few weeks after their arrival until fully vaccinated. For those destined to be outdoor cats, the transition from using a litter tray to soil in the garden can be eased by filling the tray with sterilised soil.

To prevent damage to the furniture, scratching posts should be provided even if the kitten is destined to be an outdoor cat. It should be encouraged to use the posts when caught scratching at inappropriate surfaces. It may be necessary to help it manually to scratch at the post by holding the paws against it and raking the claws gently downwards.

As discussed in Chapter 5, the critical period for learning does not stop abruptly at seven weeks. Even if a kitten is obtained at twelve weeks of age, it is vital to offer it a wide variety of experiences, both social and environmental. It should meet people of both sexes and of all ages. The owner should interact with it frequently, both handling it and playing with it. Until it can be safely allowed out of doors, owners should walk around the garden with it in their arms to accustom it early to the sights, sounds and smells there. The owner should observe her kitten's reactions and, if it seems fearful of a particular person or situation, efforts should be made immediately to desensitize it (see page 53).

## Acquiring an adult cat

There is no reason why a cat which has been a problem free pet in one household should not make a satisfactory pet in another. Also, a cat whose behaviour has posed a problem in one house where, for example, there are other cats may become a trouble free pet in another where the situation is different: for example where it is the only cat. When a cat joins a household as an adult, similar precautions should be taken as when moving house (see page 74).

Elderly owners are often understandably worried that their pet will have no home if they die or have to go into hospital. Organisations now exist (see Useful Addresses) which find adoptive or foster homes for pets in such circumstances and owners acquiring a new cat may gain extra satisfaction from the knowledge that they are helping both a cat and another person in this way.

Feral cats, especially if adopted as adults, seldom make satisfactory pets. The risk of disease (e.g.FeLV) should also be considered if a feral cat is encouraged to mix with resident cats. Its interests are usually best served by consistently putting out food for it at some distance from the house. It may also be offered shelter and bedding in an outhouse to which it can gain free access. If possible it should be trapped and sterilised: local cat rescue societies can often help with equipment and expertise. After sterilisation, male cats in particular may become more friendly; they may even be willing to adopt a lifestyle as indoor pets. Those which remain shy should be cared for as outdoor pets.

## Owning more than one cat

Cat lovers frequently own more than one cat in order to increase their own enjoyment. There can also be advantages from the cat's point of view in being part of a multi-cat household. As discussed in Chapter 3, cats are often more social than is commonly supposed and they can benefit from the company and stimulation provided by another cat, particularly if they are indoor cats or if the owners are out all day. Owners should realise, however, that the likelihood of problems such as aggression between cats often increases with the number of cats in a household.

The best way of avoiding problems of social incompatibility is to acquire two or more cats as kittens from the same litter. Otherwise, when introducing a cat or kitten into a household with a resident cat, precautions should be taken to avoid antagonism. Similar considerations apply when there is a resident dog. Ideally, the new kitten or cat should be housed initially in an indoor pen: this allows the resident cat to become accustomed to its presence and smell. It also protects the new arrival from attack or over enthusiastic attempts at greeting. Over the course of about a week, the pen should be moved from room to room to establish the new cat's occupancy throughout the house. In addition, damp litter used by the new cat can be placed in the resident cat's tray and vice versa to encourage acceptance of each other's scent. The cats can also be fed alongside each other, separated by the bars of the pen. The first of the free introductions should be carefully supervised with one or both cats restrained by hand; harnesses can be useful here if the cats have become accustomed to wearing them beforehand.

## Cats and babies

Couples are sometimes concerned about the possible reaction of their cat to the arrival of a new baby. A few cats may indeed show aggression towards the baby, because they perceive it either as strange and threatening or as a competitor for the owners' attention. Although the risk is overestimated by many worried parents, there is also the theoretical possibility that the cat may inadvertently harm the baby by sitting or sleeping on it; it might also attempt to play with the baby. Until he or she is old enough to be safe from such dangers, the cat should not be left alone with a new baby.

In addition, cats may begin to spray urine or eliminate indoors when a baby arrives. The baby's clothes or equipment may be targeted. Usually such responses are transient, ceasing after a few weeks as the cat becomes accustomed to the baby.

If the cat is one which frequently demands the owners' attention, the owners should restructure the relationship between themselves and the cat before the baby arrives. The cat should become accustomed to the owner rejecting its advances and to interactions being initiated by the owner. In all cases, it is important that the cat, while being safely restrained, should be allowed to smell the baby and its equipment, especially nappies with their strong scent. In general, the cat should receive more attention when the baby is present, but only after the baby has received attention. Contact with the baby will then be perceived as the precursor of increased attention from the owner, rather than as competition. Later, when the baby starts to crawl, the cat may again feel threatened. It is important to make sure that childproof refuges are available in every room: these are usually high places such as windowsills or cupboard tops.

## MOVING HOUSE

Many owners are aware that moving house can be a stressful experience for their cat; they are justifiably concerned that the cat may get lost in its new environment or even try to return to its old home. It is wise to take some precautions to ensure that the cat accepts and settles down in its new surroundings.

Nervous cats should be boarded in a cattery before packing up at the old house begins and they should not be brought to the new house until belongings are unpacked and furniture in position. Outdoor cats should be kept indoors in the new house for a week or so to learn the new layout and smells. Before allowing them out for the first time, they should be starved of food for about twelve hours to minimise the risk of their wandering too far from the new home and to ensure that they respond readily to sounds or calls signalling a mealtime. On the first few occasions of being allowed out they should be accompanied by the owner.

If the new home is only a short distance from the old one, it is likely that, in its explorations, the cat will encounter its familiar routes and may then keep returning to its old home. The new occupiers and their neighbours should be forewarned of this possibility and asked to refrain from encouraging the cat by feeding or petting it. Instead, they should be asked to chase the cat away and even throw a little water at it to deter it. If it persists in loitering around the old house and the owners are frequently called to collect it, they should return it to their new house by an indirect and lengthy route, in order to confuse its sense of direction. Persistent returners may have to be confined to their new home for a matter of weeks and the bond between owner and cat strengthened with frequent interaction and feeds (see Under attachment page 66).

## FURTHER READING FOR OWNERS

NEVILLE, P. (1990). *Do Cats Need Shrinks?* Sidgwick and Jackson, London.

BESSANT, C. (1992). *How to Talk to Your Cat.* Smith Gryphon, London.

# REFERENCES

ADORNO, T. W. and FENKEL-BRUNSWICK, E. (1950). *The Authoritarian Personality*. New York, Harper.

BATES, E. and MCCULLOCH, M. J. (1983). In: *New Perspectives on our Lives with Companion Animals*, (Eds. A. H. Katcher and A. M. Beck), University of Pennsylvania Press.

BATESON, P. (1987). Imprinting as a process of competitive exclusion. In: *Imprinting and cortical plasticity*, (Eds. R. Rauschecker and P. Marler) Wiley, New York.

BEADLE, M. (1977). *The Cat: History, Biology and Behaviour*. Simon and Schuster, New York.

BERRYMAN, J. C. HOWELLS, K. and LLOYD-EVANS, M. (1985). Pet owner attitudes to pets and people. *Veterinary Record* **117**, 659-61.

BIBEN, M. (1979). Predation and predatory play behaviour of domestic cats. *Animal Behaviour* **27**, 81-92.

BORCHELT, P. L. and VOITH, V. L. (1987). Aggressive behaviour in cats *Compendium on Continuing Education for the Practicing Veterinarian* **9**, 49-57.

BORCHELT, P. L. (1991). Cat elimination behaviour problems. *The Veterinary Clinics of North America* **21**, 257-265.

BRADSHAW, J. W. S. (1992). *Behaviour of the Domestic Cat*. CAB International, Wallingford,

CATANZARO, T. G. (1988). A survey on the question of how well veterinarians are prepared to predict their clients human-animal bond. *Journal of the American Veterinary Medical Association* **192**, 1707-11.

CHESLER, P. (1969). Maternal Influence in Learning by Observation in Kittens. *Science* **166**, 901-3

COOPER, L. C. and HART, B. L. (1980). Comparison of Diazepam with progestin for effectiveness in depression of spraying behaviour in cats. *Journal of the American Veterinary Medical Association* **200**, 797-801

DANTZER, R. (1983). De-arousal properties of stereotypied behaviour evidence from pituitary adrenal correlation in pigs. *Applied Animal Ethology* **10**, 244.

EGER, C. E. (1988). The treatment of urine spraying in cats by olfactory tractotomy: a safe and humane option. *Australian Veterinary Practitioner* **18**, 147-154.

EYSENCK, H. J. (1960). *The Structure of Human Personality*. Methuen, London.

FAY R. R.(1988). Comparative psychoacoustics. *Hearing Research* **34**, 295-306.

FEAVER, J. M. MENDL, M. T. and BATESON, P (1986). Variations in Domestic Cat Behaviour Towards Humans: A Paternal Effect. *Animal Behaviour* **34**, 1890-2

FEAVER J. M. MENDL, M. T. and BATESON P. (1986). A Method for Rating the Individual Distinctiveness of Domestic Cats. *Animal Behaviour* **34**, 1016-25.

FELTHOUS A. R. (1981). Childhood cruelty to cats, dogs and other animals. *Bulletin of the American Academy of Psychiatric Law* **14**, 55-69.

FOGLE B. (1991). *The Cat's Mind*. Pelham Books, London.

# REFERENCES

FOX M. W. (1974). *Understanding your Cat*. Coward, McCann and Geoghegan, New York,

HART B. L. and BARRETT R. E. (1973). Effects of castration on fighting, roaming and urine spraying in adult male cats. *Journal of the American Veterinary Medical Association* 1963, 290-292

HART B. L. (1979). Breed-specific behaviour. *Feline Practice* **9**, 10.

HART B. L. (1980). Objectionable urine spraying and urine marking in cats: evaluation of progestin treatment in gonadectomized males and females. *Journal of the American Veterinary Medical Association* **177**, 529-533.

HART B. L. (1981). Olfactory tractotomy for control of objectionable urine spraying and urine marking in cats. *Journal of the American Veterinary Medical Association* **171**, 231.

HART B. L. (1982). Neurosurgery for behavioural problems: a curiosity or the new wave? *Veterinary Clinics of North America* **12**, 707-714.

HART B. L. and COOPER L. (1984). Factors relating to urine spraying and fighting in prepubertally gonadectomized cats. *Journal of the American Veterinary Medical Association* **184**, 1255-1258.

HART B. L. and HART L. A. (1985). *Canine and feline behaviour therapy*. Lee and Febiger, Philadelphia.

HENIK R. A., OLSON P. N. and ROYCHUK R. A. W. (1985). Progestogen therapy in cats. *Compendium on Continuing Education for the Practicing Veterinarian* **7**, 132-137.

KARSH E. B. (1984). Factors influencing the socialisation of cats to people. In: *The Pet Connection*, (Eds R. Anderson, B. L. Hart and L. A. Hart), University of Minnesota Press.

KARSH E. B. and TURNER D. C. (1988). The Human-Cat Relationship. In: *The Domestic Cat: The Biology of Its Behaviour.* (Eds. D. C. Turner and P. Bateson), Cambridge University Press.

KENSHALO D. R. (1964). The temperature sensitivity of furred skin of cats. *Journal of Physiology.* **172**, 439.

KERBY G. and MACDONALD D. W. (1988). Cat society and the consequences of colony size. In: *The Domestic Cat: The Biology of Its Behaviour.* (Eds. D. C. Turner and P. Bateson), Cambridge University Press.

KERTSIN I. T. (1968). Pavlov's Concept of Experimental Neurosis and Abnormal Behaviour in Animals. In: *Abnormal Behaviour in Animals*, (Ed. M. W. Fox) Saunders, Philadelphia,

KOMTEBEDDE J. and HAUPTMAN J .(1990). Bilateral ischiocavaernosus myectomy for chronic urine spraying in castrated male cats. *Veterinary Surgery* **19**, 293-296.

KUO Z. Y. (1930). The Genesis of the Cats Response to the Rat. *Journal of Comparative Psychology* **11**, 1-35.

KUO Z. Y. (1960). Studies on the basic factors in animal fighting. 7. Inter-species co-existence in mammals. *Journal of Genetic Psychology* **97**, 211-25.

LANDSBERG, G. M. (1991). Feline destruction and the effects of declawing. *Veterinary Clinics of North America* **21**, 265-279.

LEDGER R. (1993). Factors influencing the responses of kittens to humans and novel objects. Unpublisheded MSc Thesis, University of Edinburgh.

# REFERENCES

LUESCHER U. A., MCKEOWN D. B. and HALIP J. (1991). Stereotypic or obsessive-compulsive disorders in dogs and cats. *Veterinary Clinics of North America* **21**, 401-415.

LEYHAUSEN, P. (1965). Communal organization of solitary mammals. *Proceedings of the Symposium of Zoological Society of London* **14**, 249-263.

MACDONALD D. W., APPS P. J., CARR G. M. and KERBY G. (1987). The social behaviour of a group of semi-dependent farm cats, Felis catus: a progress report. *Carnivore Genetics Newsletter*, **3**, 256-268.

MARDER A. R. (1991). Psychotropic drugs and behavioural therapy. *Veterinary Clinics of North America* **21**, 329-342.

MEIER G. W. (1961). Infantile Handling and Development in Siamese Kittens. *Journal of Comparative Physiology and Psychology* **54**, 284-6.

MERTENS C. and SHAR R. (1988). Practical Aspects of Research on Cats. In: *The Domestic Cat: The Biology of Its Behaviour.* (Eds. D. C. Turner and P. Bateson), Cambridge University Press.

MESSANT P. and HORSEFIELD S. (1985). Pet population and the pet-owner bond. In: The Human-Pet Relationship. *Proceedings of the International Symposium. Austrian Academy of Biological Sciences* IEMT, Vienna.

MOELK M. (1979). The level of friendly approach behaviour in the cat. In: *Advances in the Study of Behaviour.* Vol 10. (Eds. J. S. Rosenblatt, R. A. Hinde, C. Beer and M. Busnel, Academic Press, New York.

NEVILLE P. (1990) *Do Cats Need Shrinks?* Sidgewick and Jackson, London.

NEVILLE P. (1991). *In: Annual Report of the Association of Pet Behaviour Counsellors.*

NILSSON B. Y. and SKOGLUND C. R. (1965). The tactile hairs on the cat's foreleg. *Acta Physiologica Scandinavica* **65**, 364.

O'FARRELL V. (1992). *Manual of Canine Behaviour, 2nd edition.* BSAVA Publications, Cheltenham.

O'FARRELL V. (1994) *Dog's Best Friend.* Methuen, London.

OLM D. and HOUPT K. A. (1988). Feline house soiling problems. *Applied Animal Behaviour Science* **20**, 335-345.

PAVLOV I. P. (1927). *Conditioned Reflexes.* Oxford University Press.

RANDI E. and RAGLI B., 1991. Genetic variability and biochemical systematics of domestic and wild-cat populations (Felis sylvestris: felidi). *Journal of Mammology* **72**, 79-88.

RITVO H. (1985). Animal pleasures: popular zoology in 18th and 19th century England. *Harvard Library Bulletin,* **33**, 239-79.

ROSENBLATT J. S. (1971). Suckling and home orientation in the kitten: a comparative development study. In: *The Biopsychology of Development.* (Eds. E. Tobach, L.R. Aronson and E. Shaw E.), Academic Press, New York.

RUSHDEN J., SCHOUTEN W., DE PASSILLE A. M. B. et. al. (1990). Are stereotypies in pigs a coping mechanism? *Proceedings of the Society of Veterinary Ethologists* **4**.

SCHARFF D. E. and SCHARFF J. S. (1991). *Object relations couple therapy.* New Jersey, Aronson

# REFERENCES

SEITZ P. F. D .(1959). Infantile experience and adult behaviour in animal subjects. 2. Age of Separation from the mother and adult behaviour in the cat. *Psychosomatic Medicine* **21**, 353-78.

SERPELL J. A. (1988). The domestication and history of the cat. In: *The Domestic Cat: The Biology of Its Behaviour.* (Eds. D. C. Turner and P. Bateson), Cambridge University Press.

SHERMAN S. M. (1973). Visual field defects in monocularly and binocularly deprived cats. *Brain Research* **49**, 25.

SIMONSEN M. (1979). Effects of Maternal Malnourishment, Development and Behaviour in Successive Generations in the Rat and Cat. In: *Malnutrition, Environment and Behaviour.* (Ed. D. A. Levitsky), Cornell University Press.

SMITH B. A. and JANSEN G. R. (1977). Maternal Undernutrition in the Feline: Behavioural Sequelae. *Nutrition Reports International*, **16**, 513-26.

SMART R. G. (1965). Conflict and Conditioned Aversive Stimuli in the Development of Experimental Neuroses. *Canadian Journal of Psychology* **19**, 208-223.

TABOR R. (1983). *The Wildlife of the Domestic Cat.* Arrow Books, London.

THOMAS F. E. and DEWALD L. (1977). Experimental Neurosis: Neuro-Physiological Analysis. In: *Psychopathology: Experimental Models* (Eds. J. D. Maser and M. E. P. Seligman. Freeman, San Francisco,

TURNER D. C., FEAVER J. M., MENDL M. T. and BATESON P. (1986). Variations in domestic cat behaviour towards humans: a paternal effect. *Animal Behaviour* **34**, 1890-1892.

TURNER D. C. and STAMMBACH-GEERING I. (1990-91). Owner assessment and the ethology of human-cat relationship. In: *Pets, benefits and practice.* (Ed I.H. Burger) BVA Publications, London.

TURNER D. C.'s (1991). The ethology of the human-cat relationship. *Schweizer Archivfur Tierheilkunde.* **133**, 63-70.

VOITH V. L. (1984). Human/animal relationships. In: *Nutrition and Behaviour of Dogs and Cats.* (Ed. R.S. Anderson ). Pergammon Press, Oxford.

VOITH V. L. and BORCHELT P. L. (1986). Social Behaviour of Domestic Cats. *Compendium on Continuing Education for the Practicing Veterinarian* **8**, 637-644.

VOITH V. L .(1989). *Behavioural disorders. In: Textbook of Veterinary internal medicine.* (Ed S. Ettinger) W. B. Saunders, Philadelphia.

WALKER V. and BEECH HH R. (1969). Mood state and the ritualistic behaviour of obsessional patients. *British Journal of Psychiatry.* **115**, 1261-1268.

WATT S. L. (1991). *Companion animal cruelty.* Unpublished MSC Thesis. University of Edinburgh

WILBUR R. H. (1976). Pet ownership and animal control, social and psychological attitudes. *1975 report to National Conference on Dog and Cat Control*, Denver, Colorado

WILSON V. J. and MELVILLE JONES G. (1979). *Mammalian Vestibular Physiology.* Plenum Press, New York.

WILSOM M., WARREN J. M. and ABBOT L. (1965). Infantile stimulation, activity and learning by cats. *Child Development* **36**, 843-53.

WOLPE J. (1952). Experimental neurosis as learned behaviour. *British Journal of Psychology*, **43**, 243-268.

# USEFUL ADDRESSES

**Information:**

Association of Pet Behaviour Counsellors
257 Royal College Street
LONDON
NW1 9LU

Feline Advisory Bureau
235 Upper Richmond Road
LONDON
SW15 6SN
Tel: 081 789 9553

Companion Animal Behaviour Therapy
Study Group
Mr. D. Mills B.V.Sc. M.R.C.V.S.
74 Glen Park Avenue,
Mutley,
Plymouth
PL4 6BE

**Rescue, Fostering and Adoption**

Pet Fostering Service (Scotland)
Tel: 041 332 7910

Cinnamon Trust - Pet fostering and adoption
for the elderly and terminally ill.
Poldarves Farm
Trescowe Common
Germoe
PENZANCE
Cornwall TR20 9RX
Tel: 0736 850291

Cats Protection League
17 Kings Road
HORSHAM
W. Sussex RH13 5PP
Tel: 0403 61947

Society for Companion Animal Studies
7 Botanic Crescent Lane
GLASGOW G20 8AA
Tel: 041 945 2088

Governing Council of the Cat Fancy
4-6 Penel Orlieu
BRIDGEWATER
Somerset TA6 3PG

International Society for Anthrozoology
Dept. of Biology
University of Southampton
Bassett Crescent East
SOUTHAMPTON
Hants SO9 3TU
Tel: 0703 59500 ext 4254

**Equipment suppliers:**

For cat muzzles, kitten pens, carrying baskets,
handling equipment etc:

Mikki Pet Products
211-213 High Town Road
Luton
Bedfordshire LU2 0VZ
Tel: 0582 20428   Fax: 0582 455728

# INDEX

# INDEX

# LIST OF B.S.A.V.A. PUBLICATIONS

## THE JOURNAL OF SMALL ANIMAL PRACTICE

An International Journal Published Monthly     Editor W. D. Tavernor, BVSc, PhD, FRCVS
Fifteen Year Cumulative Index published 1976
*Available by post from:*     B.S.A.V.A. Administration Office, Kingsley House, Church Lane,
Shurdington, Cheltenham, Gloucestershire GL51 5TQ

**Manual of Parrots, Budgerigars and other Psittacine Birds**
Edited by C. J. Price, MA, VetMB, MRCVS
*B.S.A.V.A. Publications Committee 1988*

**Manual of Laboratory Techniques**
Third Edition
Edited by D. L. Doxey, BVM&S, PhD, MRCVS
and M. B. F. Nathan, MA, BVSc, MRCVS
*B.S.A.V.A. Publications Committee 1989*

**Manual of Anaesthesia for Small Animal Practice**
Third Revised Edition
Edited by A. D. R. Hilbery, BVetMed, MRCVS
*B.S.A.V.A. Publications Committee 1992*

**Manual of Radiography and Radiology in Small Animal Practice**
Edited by R. Lee, BVSc, DVR, PhD, MRCVS
*B.S.A.V.A. Publications Committee 1989*

**Manual of Small Animal Neurology**
Edited by S. J. Wheeler, BVSc, CertVR, PhD, MRCVS
*B.S.A.V.A. Publications Committee 1989*

**Manual of Small Animal Dentistry**
Edited by C. E. Harvey, BVSc, DACVS, DAVD, MRCVS
and H. S. Orr, BVSc, DVR, MRCVS
*B.S.A.V.A. Publications Committee 1990*

**Manual of Small Animal Endocrinology**
Edited by M. F. Hutchinson, BSc, BVMS, MRCVS
*B.S.A.V.A. Publications Committee 1990*

**Manual of Exotic Pets**
New Edition
Edited by P. H. Beynon, BVSc, MRCVS
and J. E. Cooper, BVSc, DTVM, CBiol, FIBiol, CertLAS, MRCPath, FRCVS
*B.S.A.V.A. Publications Committee 1991*

**Manual of Small Animal Oncology**
Edited by R. A. S. White, BVetMed, PhD, DVR, DACVS, FRCVS
*B.S.A.V.A. Publications Committee 1991*

**Manual of Canine Behaviour**
Second Edition
V. O'Farrell, PhD
*B.S.A.V.A. Publications Committee 1992*

**Manual of Ornamental Fish**
Edited by R. L. Butcher, MA, VetMB, MRCVS
*B.S.A.V.A. Publications Committee 1992*

**Manual of Reptiles**
Edited by P. H. Beynon, BVSc, MRCVS
J. E. Cooper, BVSc, DTVM, CBiol, FIBiol, CertLAS, MRCPath, FRCVS
and M. C. P. Lawton, BVetMed, CertVOphthal, CertLAS, CBiol, FIBiol, FRCVS
*B.S.A.V.A.. Publications Committee 1992*

**Manual of Small Animal Dermatology**
Edited by P. H. Locke, BVSc, MRCVS,
R. G. Harvey, BVSc, DVD, CBiol, MIBiol, MRCVS
and I. S. Mason, BVetMed, CertSAC, PhD, MRCVS
*B.S.A.V.A. Publications Committee 1993*

**Manual of Small Animal Ophthalmology**
Edited by S. M. Petersen-Jones, DVetMed, DVOphthal, MRCVS
and S. M. Crispin, MA, VetMB, BSc, PhD, DVA, DVOphthal, MRCVS
*B.S.A.V.A. Publications Committee 1993*

**Manual of Small Animal Arthrology**
Edited by R. W. Collinson, BVMS, CertSAO, MRCVS
J. E. F. Houlton, MA, VetMB, DVR, DSAO, MRCVS
*B.S.A.V.A. Publications Committee 1994*

**Manual of Feline Behaviour**
V. O'Farrell, PhD
P. Neville, BSc
Edited by C. St. C. Ross, BVM&S, MRCVS
*B.S.A.V.A. Publications Committee 1994*

**An Introduction to Veterinary Anatomy and Physiology**
By A. R. Mitchell, MA, VetMB, MRCVS
and P. E. Watkins, MA, VetMB, DVR, MRCVS
*B.S.A.V.A. Publications Committee 1989*

**Proceedings of the B.S.A.V.A. Symposium "Improved Healthcare in Kennels and Catteries"**
Edited by P. H. Beynon, BVSc, MRCVS
*B.S.A.V.A. Publications Committee 1991*

**Practice Resource Manual**
Edited by D. A. Thomas, BVetMed, MRCVS
*B.S.A.V.A. Publications Committee 1991*

**Members Information Service**
Edited by D. A. Thomas, BVetMed, MRCVS
*B.S.A.V.A. Publications Committee 1993*

**Practical Veterinary Nursing**
Third Edition
Edited by G. M. Simpson, BVM&S, MRCVS
*B.S.A.V.A. Publications Committee 1994*

**Small Animal Formulary**
B. J. Tennant, BVSc, PhD, CertVR, MRCVS
*B.S.A.V.A. Publications Committee 1994*

**B.S.A.V.A. VIDEO 1** (VHS and BETA)
**Radiography and Radiology of the Canine Chest**
Presented by R. Lee, BVSc, DVR, PhD, MRCVS
Edited by M. McDonald, BVSc, MRCVS
*B.S.A.V.A. Publications Committee 1983*

### *AVAILABLE FROM BOOKSELLERS*

**Canine Medicine and Therapeutics**
Third Edition
Edited by E. A. Chandler, BVetMed, FRCVS
D. J. Thompson, OBE, BA, MVB, MRCVS
J. B. Sutton, MRCVS
and C. J. Price, MA, VetMB, MRCVS
*Blackwell Scientific Publications 1991*

**Feline Medicine and Therapeutics**
Second Edition
Edited by E. A. Chandler, BVetMed, FRCVS
C. J. Gaskell, BVSc, PhD, DVR, MRCVS,
and R. M. Gaskell, BVSc, PhD, MRCVS
*Blackwell Scientific Publications 1994*

**An Atlas of Canine Surgical Techniques**
Edited by P. G. C. Bedford, PhD, BVetMed, FRCVS
*Blackwell Scientific Publications 1984*

**Jones's Animal Nursing**
Fifth Edition
Edited by D. R. Lane, BSc, FRCVS
*Pergamon Press 1989*